Testimonials

April 14, 1986

"A friend of mine loaned me Stretching Scientifically. I started to read it, and could not put it down! I feel like maybe there is a chance for me now. I am 40 years old and have been involved in Tae Kwon Do for **six** years—I work very hard but after six years, my kicks are still low—gut high—with fair power.

But I have been doing much of my hard work backwards!

Thank you so much for writing your book."—Victor Roggio, St. Peters, Pennsylvania.

September 26, 1986

"I have been using your technique consistently. Yours is the only technique that has actually increased my stretch, that I have tried in the last four years."—Victor Roggio, St. Peters, Pennsylvania.

"This book has greatly improved my flexibility and was a great benefit to my students as well."—John Vest, Scottsburg, Indiana.

". . . I have never been able to display my maximum range of motion without thoroughly warming up, a process lasting some 30 to 45 minutes, and muscles would always be limited in mobility early in the morning. Using your method, I am able to achieve the same stretch in only five minutes, and perform with maximal range of motion even in the morning! . . . stretching is no longer a tedious task. Stretching Scientifically is, without doubt, the most effective, efficient and safest method of stretching. . . ."—Mr. H. D. Palfrey, Gillingham, England.

"This scientific method definitely works. Thanks a lot!!!"—Ken Nero, Silver Spring, Maryland.

"It's definitely the most comprehensive thing out on flexibility."—Kirk Peck, Boulder, Colorado.

"I am very impressed with the book and tape Stretching Scientifically. The 'two' is what I really needed."—Rick Manglinong, So. Lake Tahoe, California.

Stretching Scientifically

A Guide to Flexibility Training

by Thomas Kurz, M.Sc.

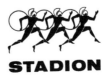

STADION

Stretching Scientifically
A Guide to Flexibility Training
by Thomas Kurz, M.Sc.

Published by:

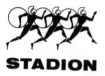

STADION

Stadion Publishing Company
a division of Stadion Enterprises
Post Office Box 6009-165
Cypress, CA 630-0009, U.S.A.

Copyright © 1987 by Thomas Kurz
  Printed in the United States of America
  Library of Congress Catalog Card Number 87-61431
  ISBN 0-940149-28-1 (paper trade)
  ISBN 0-940149-26-5 (library binding)

Cover and Book Design by Eva Chodkiewicz-Swider
Photography by Jerzy Tomasik and Alexander Calzatti

I dedicate this book to Antoni Zagorski and late Tadeusz Sadowski. Without their help it would have never been written.

About the author

Before coming to U.S.A., Thomas Kurz studied physical education in one of the top East European institutions preparing coaches, teachers of physical education and rehabilitation specialists.

He studied for five years at AWF (Academy of Physical Education) in Warsaw. While still a student he was appointed assistant coach of the students judo team. Due to the nature of his studies he competed in several Olympic sports. This contributed to his expertise in the field of methodology of sports and physical education, the expertise so evident in his work with his students as well as in this book.

Mark Bazylko, M.Sc.

Acknowledgments

Everything I know about physical education, sports and training, I have learned from teachers at AWF. They taught me the most modern (if something so advanced can be called merely modern) methods of training. To them and all East Block P.E. teachers and coaches this book is nothing new, because all I did was to put in writing a small portion of what they have been teaching since many years. I am specially grateful to Dr. Antoni Olszowski, the prorector of AWF in Warsaw, for bringing to my and my fellow students attention the importance of methodology of physical education and sports.

Preface

In this book you will find all the information about flexibility training that you need to succeed in sports. First edition of this book was a great success. Several readers wrote me about the gains they had made thanks to my instruction. There were readers though, that either had difficulty understanding these instructions, fitting the exercises into their training, or after initial rapid gains reached level well short of their goal (and their potential too) and could not progress any more. Using the feedback from all these readers I completely rewrote the book. Now it is even more understandable and more informative. If you have read only the books and research papers on flexibility, that were published in the West, you will notice that I either use different terms writing about this subject or that familiar terms denote something else than usually. It is so because I was trained in completely different system of physical education and sport. The terms I use are direct translation of the terms used in East Block's Physical Education and Sport Methodology. Methodology of P.E. and Sport is the central subject in university courses for coaches and P.E. teachers there. Knowledge of it makes all the difference between success and failure in developing athletic skills and abilities, or simply, getting the results of exercises. Describing methods of stretching I gave as much information about correct ways of working out as possible without making this book a manual of Methodology of P.E.

TABLE OF CONTENTS

Warning—Disclaimer

I. Introduction

You most likely already know what flexibility is and what are advantages to having it developed to a high level. It is one of the essential motor qualities of an athlete. High level of flexibility helps to perform more economically in fencing, judo, wrestling, and in other sports. Certain sports require maximal development of it just for execution of their basic techniques (gymnastics, javelin throw, kickboxing). Some of our motor qualities are either inborn, like speed, or to reach exceptional level, have to be developed at certain age, like for example, balance.

Flexibility as well as strength and endurance can be brought to high values by anybody and at any time in one's life. There is no such thing as inborn flexibility—except for pathological cases.

Flexibility can be improved by doing exercises like running, swimming and weightlifting as long as your limbs go through the full range of motion. Not all athletes though can always lift weights or run middle and long distances. At some stages of training it can interfere with development of their special form. Properly chosen stretching exercises are less time and energy consuming than these indirect ways.

Apart from increasing range of movements in joints, stretching has other uses in your workout. At the beginning of the workout some stretches can be good warm-up exercises. At the end of it, stretching facilitates recovery regulating muscular tension, relieving muscle spasms and improving blood flow in muscles. It makes great cool-down exercise.

If you train rationally, good stretching method will let you have great flexibility even without a warm-up. This is essential for coaches so they can demonstrate techniques immediately when it is needed. Lack of this ability indicates that either the stretching method you use is wrong or you are chronically fatigued or both . . .

Developing great flexibility is one of the easiest tasks in athletic training. It takes little time and effort to get exceptional level of it.

Why then so many people spend hours weekly, year after year, and get such meager results? There is number of reasons for it. Some of them are:

—Wrong exercises.

—Doing even good exercises at the wrong time in a workout.

—Wrong choice of training methods of developing other athletic abilities and skills which interferes with development of flexibility as well as with total athletic development. Applying principles of methodology in training will prevent you from making any of the above mistakes. I included these principles in descriptions of stretching methods so if you follow instructions to the letter, you cannot go wrong.

Watching or participating in sports calling for generating maximum force in a movement (boxing, track and field—particularly throws and shot put, racquet sports, karate) you probably have noticed that before throwing a punch or hitting a ball, athletes instinctively make a movement in opposite direction, knowing that this will increase its force. A muscle works best if it can contract from optimal stretch. Ability of a muscle to contract is proportional to the length of its fibers. Longer muscle can exert force on the object (ball, shot, fist) on the longer trajectory, accelerating it more. The longer your muscles the more you can get out of them.

II. Theory

In this chapter you will learn most of the "why's" of stretching. The more you will know the better will be your choice of exercises and the likelihood of getting the results you want.

Let's start with description of body organs that decide how flexible you are.

Skeletal muscle consists of many muscle fibers (cells) arranged in parallel bundles. Muscles can grow in length and diameter, have the ability to contract and if relaxed, are very elastic. When a muscle contracts, two kinds of protein (actin and myosin) in its cells slide along one another. In the body, a muscle can be contracted to 70% or stretched to 130% of its normal resting length. Normal resting length is the length which the muscle takes up in the body in a typical resting attitude. Outside the body the muscle can be contracted to 50% of its length and stretched much more than to 130%. As a muscle is stretched beyond its normal resting length, its force of contraction gradually drops to zero at 175% of resting length. Diminishing strength of contraction is caused by decreasing amount of overlap between actin and myosin.

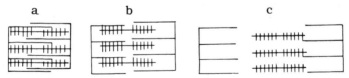

Amount of overlap of actin and myosin
a) in contracted, b) resting and c) stretched muscle.

Cutting off the flow of blood to the muscle reduces its elasticity. Flexibility improves with increased flow of blood in stretched muscles.

Whole muscle is encased in a connective tissue sheath (epimisium), bundles and even single cells are also surrounded by the same tissue (perimisium and endomisium). Tension generated by muscle cells is transferred to the fibers of connective tissue.

Tendons are cordlike extensions of this tissue. Collagen fibers, a major element of connective tissue, have great strength, no elasticity and cannot contract. These fibers are arranged in wavy bundles allowing motion until the slack of these bundles is taken up. Extension of a tendon beyond four percent of its length causes irreversible deformation. Improper use of isometric or eccentric tensions can put too much stress on collagen fibers damaging them and causing muscle soreness—a result of disintegration of collagen and release of hydroxyproline, one of its components, into the muscle. With age molecules of collagen change becoming more rigid and this is reflected in general body stiffness.

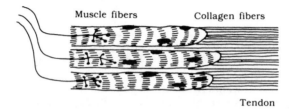

Collagen fibers surrounding muscle fibers at their junction with the tendon.

Joint capsule is a connective tissue sleeve completely surrounding each movable joint. Immobilization for a few weeks causes chemical changes in collagen fibers of the joint capsule that will restrict your flexibility.

Ligaments holding your joints together are made primarily of collagen fibers. They have more elastic fibers, made of protein elastin, than do tendons. Stretching ligaments leads to loose-jointness and can be effectively applied only with children. In adults, age related increase in rigidity of collagen fibers makes any stretches aimed at elongating ligaments hazardous. When children stretch ballistically or statically, their muscles do not contract as strongly as adult's and ligaments can be stretched. If a ligament is stretched more than six percent of its normal length—it tears. There is no need to stretch ligaments to perform even the most spectacular karate or gymnastic techniques. Natural range of motion is sufficient.

Bone is a dynamic, living tissue made of crystals of calcium and phosphorus associated with collagen fibers. Exercises can change density and shape of bones. The forms of joint surfaces, covered by glasslike, smooth and elastic cartilage, change in the long-term process of exercise, e.g., dynamic stretching. Depending on the amount of stress (exercise), bones and joints can adapt to it or be destroyed by it.

Here are some simple tests to convince you that the structure of joints and length of ligaments does not keep you from doing splits:

Front split. If the angle between front and rear leg is less than 180 degrees with front leg straight, flex its knee and see what happens. . .

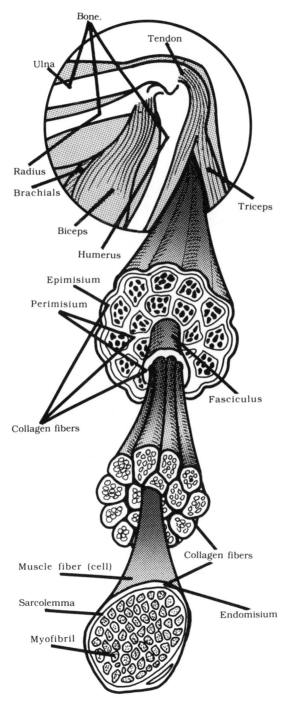

Cross-section through a skeletal muscle.

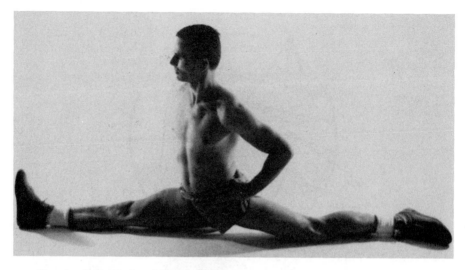

Front split with front leg straight.

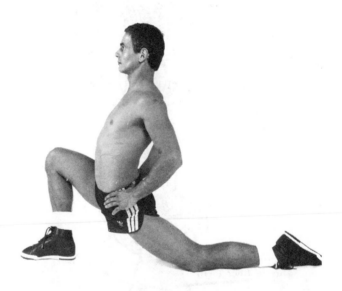

Deep lunge. The knee of the front leg is flexed and the angle between thighs is 180 degrees.

If you started to stretch past the age when elongating ligaments was possible, you probably have difficulty with touching the ground with front of the thigh of the rear leg in this split. What keeps you from doing it is usually not a muscle but a ligament (lig. iliofemorale) running in front of your hip joint. It is tightened by extension of the hip (posterior tilting of the pelvis or moving the thigh to the back while keeping the pelvis straight). Flexing the hip (tilting the pelvis forwards or moving the thigh to the front) relaxes this ligament. To achieve a nice, flat split you need to stretch the hamstring of the front leg and the muscles of lower back so you can tilt pelvis forwards while keeping the trunk upright.

To make sure that the muscles in front of your thigh are not exceptionally short do this test: Lie on a table, on your back, with your lower legs hanging over the edge. Pull one leg, with its knee flexed, toward your chest. Keep your back flat on the table. If the other leg, left lying on the table, is lifted by this movement before the angle between thighs reaches 120 degrees, your quadriceps needs some stretching.

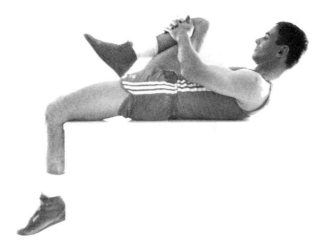

Quadriceps length test.

Side split. Person unable to do a complete split can bring one of the thighs into the position it would have in relation to the hip in the split, or at least get it much closer to this position than when spreading both legs at the same time. No muscles run from one leg to another. If you can do one half of the split, only reflexive contraction of the muscles prevents you from doing a complete split with equal ease. Please note that doing side split we do not only spread legs sideways but also tilt pelvis forwards (push buttocks to the rear). In side split with feet pointing up, the pelvis is kept straight but the thighs rotate outwards. Alignment of hips and thighs in both types of side split is the same. You cannot do this split without either rotating thighs outwards or tilting the pelvis forwards. This forward tilt (hip flexion) unwinds capsular ligaments of the hip, among them the pubofemoral ligament that resists excessive abduction. Spreading the legs without these additional movements twists and tightens ligaments of the hip and jams the thigh bones against your pelvis.

The amount of outside rotation of femur in the hip decides about the quality of your side split. It is limited by gluteus medius, gluteus minimus, psoas maior and the posterior belly of adductor magnus, the muscles rotating the thigh inside. Normally adductors pull the thigh inwards and rotate it outwards, but if the thigh is rotated outwards as much as it takes to do a side split or, so called, first ballet position; they help to rotate it inwards. It means that they are stretched also by extreme outside rotation and can limit the amount of it.

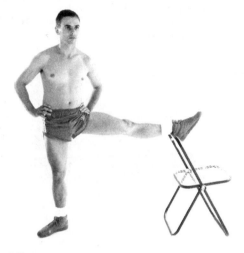

If you think that the structure of your hips will not let you do side splits, try this test . . . The leg resting on the chair is in the position it would have in a split.

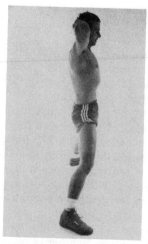

Starting position for a side split.

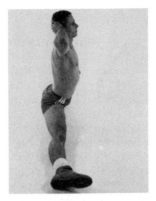

Getting into a side split legs are spread sideways and hips tilt to the rear.

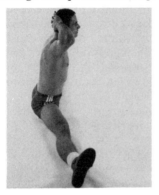

Side split with feet pointing up. The hips are straight thanks to rotation of the thighs.

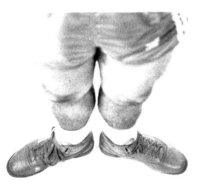 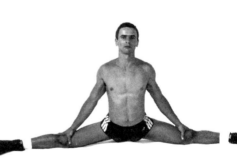

Outside rotation of the thigh in first ballet position. Nearly 90 degrees of turnout of the foot are achieved by 60 to 70 degrees of external rotation at the hip, with the remaining 20 to 30 degrees accounted for by natural outward inclination of the knee and the foot-ankle complex.
Note the relation of the angle (less than 90 degrees) in this position, to the angle (less than 180 degrees) between the thighs in a side split.

In above examples, relieving tension of muscles around the joint increases its range of motion. It means that only muscular tension prevents you from doing splits. Muscular tension has two components: tension generated by the contractile elements (muscle fibers) and the tension, present even in an inactive, denervated muscle, exerted by the connective tissues associated with it.

The nervous system regulates tension and thus length of your muscles by influencing the contractile element. Several nerve cells receive signals from and send signals to each muscle. Nerve cells receiving the signals are called afferent or sensory neurons. Directly or through other neurons they contact nerve cells that send signals to the muscles. The cells whose axons (nerve fibers) conduct signals to the muscles are called motoneurons or efferent neurons. Their cell bodies are located in the spinal cord or in the brainstem. Other neurons contact and influence motoneurons. Some can stimulate the motoneurons, which causes contraction of muscle fibers innervated by them, some can inhibit (block) motoneurons causing relaxation of muscle fibers. When motoneurons of one set of muscles are stimulated, motoneurons of muscles opposing them are inhibited. This is called reciprocal inhibition. It allows you to move. Neurons causing contraction of muscles are called motoneurons Alpha.

Within a muscle are embedded muscle spindles. They consist of a special kind of muscle fibers that can contract only at their ends. In their central part are located stretch receptors. There are two kinds of them: one responding only to the magnitude of the stretch, another to both the magnitude and the speed of stretching. Muscle spindles in a stretched muscle send signals reaching motoneuron Alpha and cause it to send impulses to the muscle. Resulting contraction lowers stimulation of the spindles.

Motoneurons Gamma are located in spinal cord, close to motoneurons Alpha. These neurons regulate tension of muscle spindles, so if the whole muscle is contracted, the spindle can adjust and still be able to detect changes in muscle length.

The brain through descending pathways (nerve fibers conducting impulses downwards from the brain) affects similarly motoneurons Alpha and Gamma, but Gamma are more sensitive.

Descending pathways, motoneuron Gamma, spindle muscle fibers, stretch receptor in this spindle, sensory neuron innervating it, and motoneuron Alpha are collectively called Gamma loop. Its activity measures and influences the length of the muscle. Thanks to it the same weight can be supported by different lengths of a muscle or the same length can support different weights. When a muscle is stretched, for example, by tapping its tendon like in testing knee-jerk reflex, receptors in spindles send impulses that through synapses reach motoneurons Alpha, stimulating contraction of this muscle and its synergists. The same impulse sent by stretch receptors inhibit muscles antagonistic to it, and your leg kicks. This is the mechanism of knee-jerk reflex. Every stretch causes a tension preventing further stretching. Gamma loop regulates sensitivity of muscle spindles for stretching. If, because of lowered tonus, insufficient amount of impulses comes from stretch receptors, Gamma loop compensates for it making the muscle shorter. This is why we are so stiff after waking up.

Apart from Gamma loop, muscular tension is regulated by Golgi organs and Renshaw cells.

Golgi organs are located in the tendon at its junction with the muscle. The contracting muscle pulls on the tendon causing Golgi organs to fire impulses in relation to the force of contraction. This stops flow of impulses from motoneuron Alpha to the muscle (isometric stretching is based on this fact). Some Golgi organs have high thresholds and act as a safety feature in case of excessive contraction or excessive stretching. The rest of Golgi organs having lower threshold supplies motor centers with information about tension of the muscle. The ones that have high threshold are the ones causing greatest relaxation. Golgi organs may also influence motoneurons Gamma.

Renshaw cells are small nerve cells located close to motoneurons Alpha. They are connected through synapses with motoneurons and are activated by the impulses that these motoneurons send to muscle fibers. Renshaw cells, through their axons synapse back on the motoneurons that activate them and on others. Impulses from Renshaw cells inhibit motoneurons. This circuit regulates frequency of impulses received by muscles and keeps them from making contractions too strong. Motoneurons Alpha responsible for static tension are more easily inhibited by Renshaw cells than the ones responsible for dynamic movements.

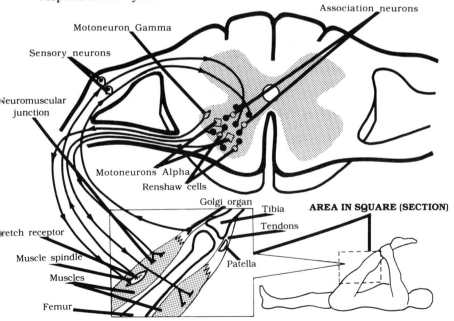

Structures and nerve pathways involved in control of muscle at the level of its corresponding segment of spinal cord.

Your kinesthetic or muscle sense is served by more than the two already described kinds of receptors (muscle spindle and Golgi organ).

Pacinian corpuscles, rapidly adapting receptors, are found in skin and sheaths of muscles and tendons. In skin they detect vibrations, in other organs also pressure.

Ruffini endings, slowly adapting receptors, sense pressure.

Three kinds of receptors are located in capsules of your joints:

—Free nerve endings signal joint pain.

—Ruffini endings, slowly adapting, scattered throughout the joint capsule, sense the position of the joint.

—Paciniform endings, rapidly adapting to stimuli, are sensitive to the direction and speed of motion.

Combined input from all receptors influences reflexive reactions to changes in body position and tension. Reflexes are never as simple as the oversimplified description of a knee-jerk. Usually the whole body responds to any stimulus. Remember the test where you could see if bones and ligaments of your hips will let you do a side split? There is no muscle or a ligament running from one thigh to another, yet, without some training, you cannot do a complete side split! When you spread both legs at the same time, reflexive contraction of muscles on both sides of the body gets in your way. Our reflexes are so arranged as to be useful in normal circumstances and when your legs slide sideways, tension of adductors and their synergists on both sides of the body is needed to maintain your posture.

So much for reflexive regulation of muscular tension. Now let's talk about its voluntary control by the brain.

The Proprioceptive-Cerebellar System. Some of the nerve fibers conducting kinesthetic information go to the cerebellum where, without you being aware of it, your tonus, coordination and balance are regulated. Other fibers go to the cerebral cortex (the outer layer of the brain, containing higher centers interpreting and correlating sensory data) and provide you with sensory data you are conscious of, or to put it even simpler; the data you feel. Neurons located in cerebral cortex contact motoneurons by descending pathways.

Direct descending pathway (pyramidal tract) consists of nerve fibers originating in cerebral cortex and ending in spinal cord, synapsing on motoneurons Alpha, Gamma and association neurons. The direct pathway governs precise, voluntary movements. Through conscious decisions to make certain movements or to contract groups of muscles we can override some of the reflexes.

In multineuronal descending pathway (extrapyramidal tract) neurons from cerebral cortex synapse through their axons with neurons in subcortical centers (nerve centers below cortex) and in the cerebellum. These latter eventually synapse either on association neurons or on motoneurons Gamma. This pathway is responsible for control of rapid movements, postural mechanisms, coordination of simultaneous movements of locomotion and coordination of fine voluntary movements with postural mechanisms. Connection between cerebellum and areas of the brain governing emotions (hippocampus, amygdala, septal areas) makes muscular tonus and coordination dependent on emotions and vice versa.

Conclusions

Muscle fibers are very elastic and in the muscle they are associated with less elastic connective tissue fibers. This is used to explain loss of flexibility solely as a result of shortening of connective tissue in and around the muscles. This shortening is to be caused by the lack of movement. It seems that there is more to it than that. Different stretching methods bring different results (dynamic stretching improves dynamic flexibility, static improves both static and dynamic flexibility) and in different time (difference between ballistic, static relaxed and isometric stretching). Possible changes to connective tissues, resulting from stretching by any of the above methods, do not explain all the differences. These differences are resulting most likely from the way given kind of exercises act upon our nervous system. Muscles are usually long enough to allow for full range of motion in joints. It is nervous control of their tension that has to be reset for the muscles to show their full length. This is why ten minutes of stretching in the morning makes using one's full range of motion possible, later in a day, without a warm-up. This is also why repeating movements not using full range of motion in joints, e.g., bicycling, certain techniques of Olympic weightlifting, pushups; causes shortening of muscles surrounding joints of the working limbs. It is a result of setting nervous control of length and tension of muscles at the values repeated most often or the strongest. Stronger stimuli are remembered better. Do you know that East Block coaches will not let gymnasts ride bicycles even though they seem to have all the flexibility they need? It is said that strenuous workouts damage slightly fibers of connective tissue in the muscles (micro-tears). Usually they heal in a day or two. Loss of flexibility is supposedly caused by these fibers healing shorter. To prevent it, static stretching after strength workouts is recommended. All this sounds very well, but the same gymnasts, that are kept from bicycling, do running with maximal accelerations to improve their specific endurance. Such running is a strenuous, intensive strength effort for leg muscles, but because in running these muscles work through full range of motion in hip and knee joints, there is no adverse effect on flexibility. If stretching after a workout would be enough, then these gymnasts could ride bicycles with the same result. The situation with pushups is very similar. If you do a couple of hundreds a day, on the floor so the muscles of your chest and shoulders contract from shortened position, no amount of static stretching will make you a pitcher or a javelin thrower.

There are two kinds of stretch receptors, one detecting magnitude and speed of stretching, the other kind magnitude only. This explains why flexibility training is speed-specific. One has to do static stretches to improve static flexibility and dynamic stretches for dynamic flexibility. This is also why it does not make sense to use static stretches as a warm-up for dynamic actions. There is considerable, but not complete transfer from static to dynamic flexibility.

Flexibility training is also position-specific. Research done by Nicolas Breit, comparing effects of stretching in supine and in erect position, shows that:

a) subjects, who trained in erect position tested better in this position than subjects who trained in supine but tested in erect position,

b) greater gains were recorded for both groups in supine test position than in erect test position. Subjects tested in erect position had to overcome extra amount of tension, in the muscles they stretched, caused by the reflexes evoked by standing and bending over.

You can use inhibiting function of Golgi organs by contracting a muscle before stretching it. This increases the amount of possible stretch. After reaching maximal stretch (maximal for you at a given stage of your training) tensing the muscle allows to hold this position and improve static strength in it. Strength increase in extreme ranges of motion, occurring after isometric stretching or after weight exercises done over the full range of motion, seems to be a result of longitudinal growth of muscle fibers.

Our coordination and flexibility depend on our emotions because of the connection between cerebellum and areas of the brain responsible for emotions. Try juggling, balancing or stretching when upset!

Yoga exercises (asanas) do not use tension in stretched position. By holding relaxed muscles in a position just short of pain and reflexive contraction, Yogis in a long-term process gradually lower the sensitivity of mechanisms regulating tension and length of the muscles. Yoga stretches seem to be a litmus test, or a sort of biofeedback monitors, telling the practitioner how proper (from Yoga point of view) his/her state of mind is.

Mental rigidity (having fixations) usually is accompanied by low level of physical flexibility.

Recap

In improving flexibility the greatest and fastest gains are made by resetting nervous control of muscle tension and length, then by special strength exercises stimulating muscle fibers to grow longer and elongating connective tissue associated with the muscle, then stretching ligaments and joint capsules and reshaping joint surfaces.

III. How to Stretch.

There are several methods of improving flexibility. In this book you will find only the safest and most efficient of them. Choice of the method or a combination of methods depends on your sport and the shape you are in.

Methods of stretching

1. Dynamic stretching: Moving parts of your body gradually increasing reach and/or speed of movement.

Perform exercises (leg raises, arm swings) in sets of eight to twelve repetitions. If after a couple of sets you feel tired—stop. Muscles tired are less elastic, which causes the decrease in amplitude of your movements. Do only the number of repetitions that you can do without diminishing the range of motion. More repetitions will set the nervous regulation of the muscles length at the level of these less than best repetitions and you may lose some of your flexibility. What is repeated more times or with greater effort will leave deeper trace in your memory! After reaching maximal range of motion in a joint in any direction of movement, you should not do many more repetitions of this movement in this workout. Even if you can maintain maximal range of motion over many repetitions, you will set unnecessarily solid memory of range of these movements. You will have to overcome these memories to make further progress.

Do not confuse dynamic stretching with ballistic stretching! In ballistic stretches momentum of a moving body or a limb is used to forcibly increase the range of motion. In dynamic stretching, as opposed to the ballistic stretching, there is no bouncing or jerky movements.

2. Static active stretching: Moving your body into a stretch and holding it there by tension of muscles-agonists in this movement. Tension of these muscles helps to relax (reciprocal inhibition) muscles opposing them, i.e., stretched.

3. Static passive stretching (Relaxed stretching): Relaxing your body into a stretch and holding it there by the weight of your body or by other external force. Slow, relaxed static stretching is useful in relieving spasms occurring in muscles healing after an injury. No stretching and no exercises at all till healing is sufficiently advanced and the doctor lets you do it!

4. Isometric stretching: Using positions similar to these in static passive stretching and adding strong tensions of the stretched muscles, you stimulate Golgi organs causing reflexive relaxations and subsequent increases of the stretch. When eventually your maximal (at this stage of training) stretch is achieved, last tension is held for up to 30 seconds or more. This increases strength of muscles in this position. Isometric stretching is the fastest stretching method. Because of the strong and long tensions it should be applied according to the same principles as other strength exercises. You should allow sufficient time for recovery after exercise depending on your shape, total volume, intensity and sequence of efforts. It may be a good idea to use isometric stretching in strength workouts, and on days when recovering from these workouts use either static relaxed stretching or replace the last, long tension in isometric stretching by just holding relaxed muscles in the final stretch.

Static forms of flexibility are fastest developed by combining isometric and static active stretching.

In your training, dynamic stretches should be used in the morning (right after waking up) as your morning stretch and later at the beginning of your workout as a part of a warm-up. Static stretches are to be done after dynamic exercises, preferably in a cool-down. If you need to display static flexibility in course of your workout or event, then these exercises should be done at the end of the warm-up.

Early morning stretching

According to Soviet and East European specialists, if you need to do movements requiring considerable flexibility with no warm-up, you ought to make the early morning stretch a part of your daily routine. The early morning stretching is done before breakfast and consists of a couple of sets of arm swings and leg raises to the front, rear and sides (dynamic stretches). Before doing these raises and swings, warm up all joints by flexing and twisting each of them. No isometric stretches are to be done in the morning. Isometric stretches may be too exhausting for your muscles to be done twice a day. You must allow sufficient time for recovery between exercises.

The whole routine can take about 30 minutes for beginners and ten to fifteen minutes for advanced. Yes, after reaching desired level of flexibility you will need less work to maintain it. You should not get tired during the morning stretching. The purpose of this stretching is to reset the nervous regulation of the length of your muscles for the rest of the day. Remember; do not work too hard because tired muscles are less elastic and if you overdo it, you defeat the purpose of this exercise.

Usually no special cool-down is needed after early morning stretching. If doing great number of repetitions you manage to considerably raise your temperature and pulse rate, slow down the pace of last sets and then spend a minute or two walking. If you have lots of time in the morning, you can also do some relaxed static stretches at the end.

Stretching in your workout

A properly designed workout plan includes the following parts:
1. General warm-up, including cardiovascular warm-up and general stretching.
2. Specific warm-up, where movements resemble closer and closer the actual subject of the workout.
3. Main part of the workout, where you realize your task.
4. Cool-down

The whole warm-up should take no more than 30 minutes. About ten minutes of this time is dedicated to stretching. Warming up you should gradually increase intensity of exercises. Toward the end of a warm-up use movements more and more resembling techniques of your sport or the task assigned for this workout.

In New York City I have seen people sitting on heaters (sic!) in order to warm up before a kickboxing workout. Warming up has to prepare all systems of the body to perform at top efficiency. It has to affect heart, blood vessels, nervous system, muscles and tendons, joints and ligaments, not just one area of the body!

Begin your warm-up with joint rotations, starting either from your toes or your fingers. Make slow circular movements till the joint moves smoothly, then move to the next one. If you start from your fingers, move on to your wrists, followed by your elbows, shoulders and the neck. Continue with twisting and bending of your trunk followed by movements in the hips, then the knees, the ankles, and finally the toes. If you start from your toes the order is reversed. The principles are: from distant joints to proximal, from one end of the body to the other, ending with the part of the body that will be used first in the next exercise. This last principle applies to all parts of a workout.

Next, five minutes of aerobic activity; for example, jogging, shadow boxing or anything having similar effect on the cardiovascular system. Flexibility improves with increased blood flow in the muscles.

After that, dynamic stretches, for example, leg raises to the front, sides and back, and arm swings. Leg raises are to be done in sets of ten to twelve repetitions per leg. Arm swings in sets of five to eight repetitions. Do as many sets as it takes to reach your maximum range of motion in any given direction. Usually, for properly conditioned athletes one set in each direction is enough.

Doing static stretches before a workout consisting of dynamic actions is counterproductive. Goals of the warm-up are: increased awareness, improved coordination, improved elasticity and contractibility of muscles, greater work efficiency of respiratory and cardiovascular systems. Static stretches, isometric or relaxed, just do not fit in here. Isometric tensions will make you tired and decrease your coordination. Passive, relaxed stretches have a calming effect and can even make you sleepy.

So much for the general warm-up. After this you can move on to the specific warm-up where choice of exercises depends on your sport and the subject of the workout. Specific warm-up blends with the main part of your workout. When the main part is over, it is time for the cool-down and final stretching. Usually only static stretches are used here. You can start with the more difficult static active stretches requiring relative "freshness". After you have achieved your maximum reach in these stretches, move on to either isometric or relaxed static stretches, or both; following isometric stretches with relaxed. Pick only one isometric stretch for one muscle group and repeat it two to five times using as many tensions per repetition (attempt) as it takes to reach the limit of mobility that you have at this stage of your training.

This is the end of your workout. If you do not participate in any sports training, but still want to stretch, just skip specific warm-up and the main part of workout. Do only stretches, starting with dynamic and ending with static.

If you follow my advice to the letter and the rest of your athletic training is run rationally, within a month you should be able to display your current level of flexibility without any warm-up. By current level of flexibility I mean the level you normally display during a workout when you are well warmed up. Of course, it is still better to warm up before exercises. Being able to do splits and high kicks does not mean that you are ready for effort. Warming up lets you perform efficiently during your workout or a sports event and speeds up the recovery afterwards. Muscles prepared for work do not gather as many chemical by-products of effort as the unprepared ones.

After required reach of motion is reached, the amount of work dedicated to flexibility may be reduced. Much less work is needed to maintain flexibility than to develop it. The amount of "maintaining" stretching will have to be increased as we age, to counter the regress of flexibility related to aging.

Flexibility in sports

Disciplines of sport can be classified according to the character of strength required in them (static, dynamic, explosive); type of effort (aerobic, anaerobic) and other factors. Similar classification can be made according to the kind and level of flexibility needed in different sports.

There are three kinds of flexibility:

—Dynamic—The ability to perform dynamic movements within full range of motion in joints.

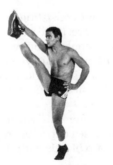
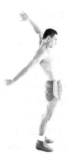

Examples of dynamic flexibility.

—Static passive—The ability to assume and maintain extended positions using one's weight (splits), strength of other than stretched limbs (lifting and holding a leg with your arm) or other external means.

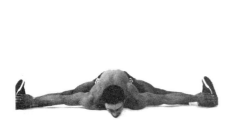
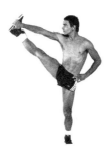

Examples of static passive flexibility.
—Static active—The ability to assume and maintain extended positions using only the tension of agonists and synergists while antagonists are being stretched, for example, lifting the leg and keeping it high without any support.

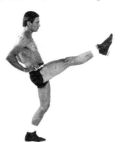
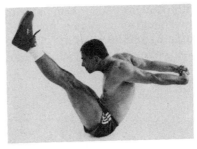

Examples of static active flexibility.
Principles of flexibility training are the same in all sports. Only required level of a given kind of flexibility vary from sport to sport.

Flexibility of an athlete is sufficiently developed when maximal reach of motion somewhat exceeds reach required in competition. This difference, between athlete's flexibility and the needs of the sport, is called "flexibility reserve" or "tensility reserve". It allows to do techniques without excessive tension and prevents injury. Achieving maximum speed in an exercise is impossible at your extreme ranges of motion, i.e., when you have no "flexibility reserve".

Training of flexibility, as well as of any other motor ability, should proceed from general, basic form, to specific—reflecting needs of particular sports. Choosing stretches you should examine your needs and requirements of your activity. For example, if you are a hurdler, you need mostly dynamic flexibility of hips, trunk and shoulders. To increase your range of motion you need to do dynamic leg raises in all directions, bends and twists of the trunk and arm swings. Your technique can be perfected by several dynamic exercises done walking or running over the hurdles. Hurdlers stretch, a static exercise, does not fit in your workout. It strains your knee by twisting it. Simple front and side splits are better for stretching your legs. Explanation that in the hurdlers stretch your position resembles the one assumed while passing the hurdle is pointless. Dynamic skills cannot be learned by using static exercises, and vice versa. The technique of running over the hurdles is better developed in motion.

Karate or kickboxing punches, blows and kicks should hit their targets with maximum speed. Some targets require fully stretched muscles of the hitting limb (in case of kicks also of the supporting leg). You know that your nervous system has a way of making sure that a stretch, particularly a sudden one, does not end abruptly causing a muscle tear. But gradually slowing down before the moment of contact will spoil the impact. You have to train your nervous system (elements of multineuronal pathway), so you can have maximal speed at the moment of contact even if it is close to maximal reach of motion in this movement. In case of kicks you can learn this skill by using your hand as a target for them. Centers in your brain, that regulate coordination and rapid movements, know about the hand, where it is and that it can stop the kick, so the leg does not have to be slowed down gradually to prevent overstretching. First develop the ability to move you limbs with moderate speed within full range of motion in joints and then do these specific, kicking drills. You should start at lower height to avoid injury from sudden contraction of rapidly stretched muscles. This exercise can only be used in a warm-up because of limited variety of kicks that can be practiced this way.

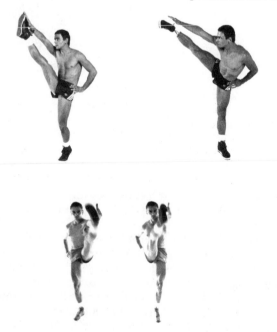

Examples of exercises developing ability to kick with maximum speed at ranges of motion required in fighting.

Fighters, relying on high kicks as their combat techniques, should spend ten to fifteen minutes in the morning on dynamic stretching of their legs. Starting slowly, they should gradually raise the legs higher. Later increase speed of movements, perhaps even use above described "hand kicking" drill. Practical experience (North Korean, Soviet Block's commando units) shows that doing actual combat kicks in this morning stretch is not necessary for being able to do them later in a day without a warm-up.

Wrestlers and judoka need specially great static strength in extreme ranges of motion to get out of holds and locks. This strength is best developed by isometric stretching and weightlifting.

Swimmers should have long hamstrings and chest muscles. When doing the breaststroke, if you go up and down in the water instead of moving just under the surface, it means that your chest muscles are too short. This shortness also causes your face to get under the surface when the arm enters the water and you want to take a breath. In the crawl short hamstrings pull your feet out of the water which makes your legwork inefficient.

You should be careful in choosing your stretches. Too much flexibility in some parts of the body can be detrimental to your sports performance. For example, in jumping, an excessively loose trunk at the moment of take-off causes scattering of forces.

Olympic weightlifters need to shorten muscles surrounding hip and knee joint for proper execution of lifts. Muscles too long let weightlifter "sink" too deep on his legs, while getting under the barbell. This makes it difficult to stand up and complete the lift.

Causes of difficulties in developing flexibility.

Here I list the most common causes of difficulties in developing athletic form in general and flexibility in particular. These are typical faults of methodology of training:

1. Wrong warm-up;—doing relaxed stretches does not significantly raise muscle temperature, increase blood flow through it, warms up joints, prepares the organism for effort.
2. Training loads too great and not enough rest cause chronic fatigue.
3. Wrong sequence of efforts in a workout and in a microcycle doubles and triples recovery time. (Microcycle is a set of workouts. It usually lasts one week.)
4. Wrong methods of teaching skills result in too many repetitions of a given exercise and chronic local fatigue.

All elements of athletic training are influencing each other. For best results in any one area of training, methods of developing all abilities have to be correct and applied taking into account each other.

The use of partners in stretching.

The practice of using partners in stretching is noneconomical and dangerous. It is noneconomical because one person in two is wasting time. The helper is neither stretching nor resting. The danger of using a partner in stretching is obvious. The partner does not feel what you feel. He or she can stretch you a bit more than you would like to. If you feel pain and let your partner know about it, by the time the partner reacts, it can be too late.

Injury prevention and flexibility.

A muscle does not have to be maximally stretched to be torn. Muscle tears are results of special combination of a sudden stretch and contraction done at the same time. Great differences of strength between opposing muscle groups as well as strength imbalance of ten per cent between the same muscle groups on both sides of the body are the main causes of injuries. Improving strength of weaker muscles is best for prevention of injuries. Also careful analysis of the form of movement may hold the key to injury prevention. Good technique feels effortless. When a particular technique injures you, revise it and try to eliminate moments when maximal tension of already stretched muscles is used to counter fast movement of relatively big mass, or to accelerate suddenly against great resistance, e.g. tears of supporting leg in kicking, hamstring tear in starting from the starting blocks. Great flexibility alone will not prevent injuries.

In the following four chapters you will find practical demonstration of principles discussed till now. Exercises are shown in a sequence that can and should be used in a workout; from dynamic movements to static ones, gradually moving from vertical to horizontal position, each exercise evolving from a previous one. You will find more than the absolutely essential number of stretches for particular groups of muscles. This way, planning a workout, you have many exercises to choose from and arrange in a methodically correct sequence suiting the subject of the workout. This is not to suggests that you should do all of them in any of your workouts. Pick one exercise for a given group of muscles. Consider facilities where workout is held and what kind of exercises precede and follow each stretch. You do not want to sit in a puddle to stretch your hamstring nor suddenly change position from standing to lying down or vice versa.

IV. Dynamic Stretching

Dynamic flexibility, the ability to perform dynamic movements within full range of motion in joints, is best developed by dynamic stretching. This kind of flexibility depends on the ability to combine relaxing of the extended muscles with contraction of the moving muscles. Besides perfecting of the intermuscular coordination, dynamic stretching improves elasticity of muscles and ligaments. Surfaces of joints change in the process of long-term flexibility training.

Dynamic flexibility is usually reduced by fatigue, so do not do dynamic stretching when your muscles are tired, unless you want to develop specific endurance and not flexibility. Stretching is most effective when carried out daily, two or more times a day. In one experiment, results of dynamic stretching for five days, twice a day (two sessions per day), thirty repetitions per session, were twice as great as the results of doing the same number of repetitions, also twice daily but every other day (one day of rest after a day of stretching). Eight to ten weeks is sufficient to achieve improvement which depends on muscle elasticity. The further increase of flexibility is insignificant, and it depends on long-term changes of bones and ligaments. This requires not intensive but rather extensive training, i.e., regular loads in course of many years.

Dynamic stretches are performed in sets, gradually increasing the amplitude of movements in a set. The number of repetitions per set is between five and twelve. Number needed to reach maximal amplitude of movement in a joint depends on the mass of muscles moving it. Reduction of amplitude is a sign to stop. Well conditioned athlete can make continuously forty or more repetitions of maximal amplitude.

Dynamic stretches should be used in your early morning stretch and as a part of general warm-up in the workout. Start movements slowly, gradually increase range and speed of movements. Do not "throw" your limbs, rather "lead" or "lift" them, controlling the movement along its entire range.

Stretches

Arms

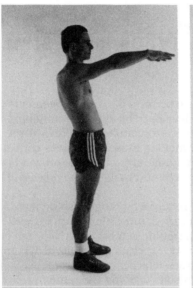 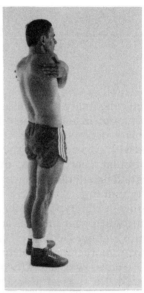

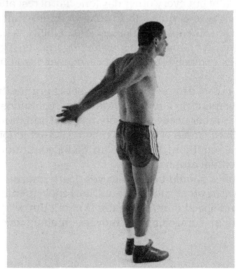

Crossing your arms in front, touch your shoulder blades with your hands, then straighten the arms and touch your hands behind your back.

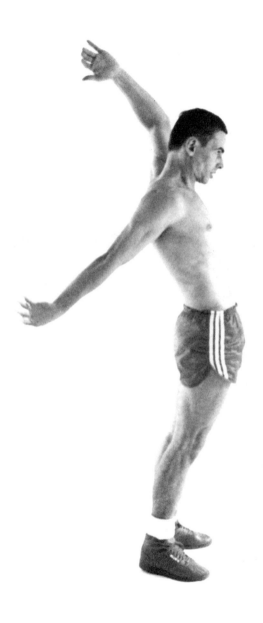

Swing your arms backwards at varying angles.

Legs

Beginners may have to start with great number of repetitions—four to five sets of ten to twelve repetitions per leg in any given direction, very slowly increasing the height at which the leg is raised. You can switch the leg after each repetition or after a set. After a month or two, you will notice that it takes less repetitions to reach maximum range of motion. Eventually one set of twelve repetitions in each direction, per leg, will be enough.

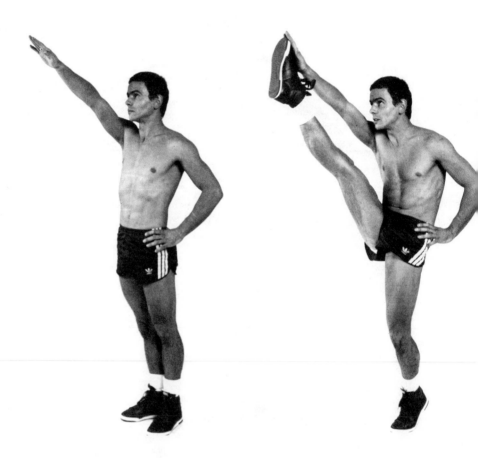

Leg raise to the front. Your hand as a target makes it easy to evaluate the progress, maintain good posture (straight trunk) and can serve as a stop for very dynamic (explosive) leg raises (see page 32). Start as low as it feels comfortable. Keep the supporting leg straight, its heel on the ground if possible.

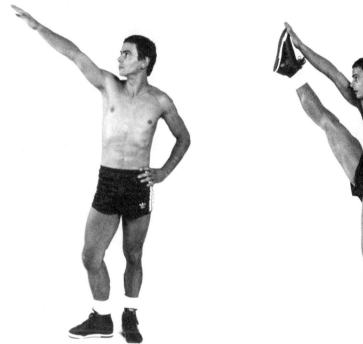
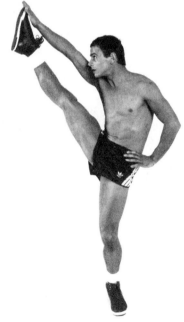

Leg raise to the side. Same as front raise, except the arm is stretched to the side and you raise your leg sideways.

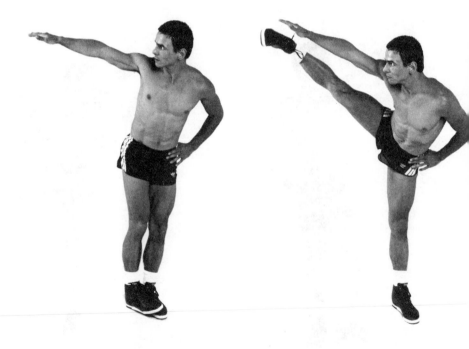

Another form of side raise. this form is useful for martial artists. Foot of the leg about to be raised points forwards and contact with the palm is made by the side of the foot. Hips have a tendency to move to the back. Try to keep them as straight as possible (do not lean forwards more than necessary). Gradually increase the height at which you keep your hand, starting at the hip level.

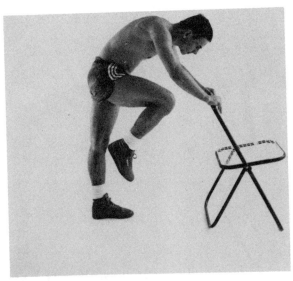

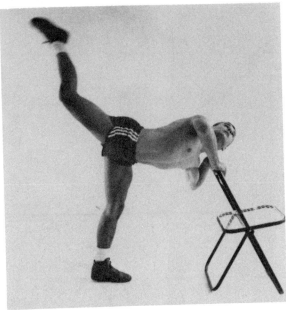

Leg raise to the back. Using any form of support at about your hip height, raise the leg as high as possible. Feel stretching in front of your thigh.

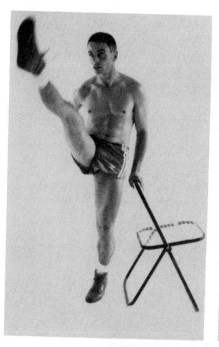 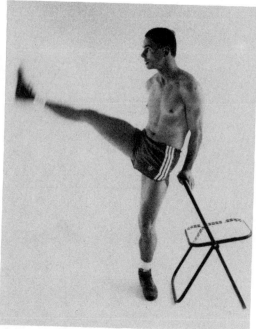

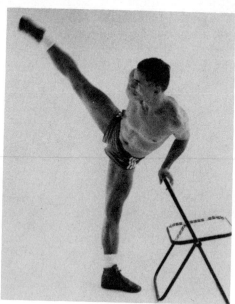

If using support lets you raise legs higher to the front and sides—use it.

Trunk

If your sports discipline requires rapid twisting and bending (with great amplitude) of the trunk, add the following set of exercises to your stretching routines. Full mobility of the trunk (joints of vertebral column) in a given direction is reached after 25-30 repetitions of a given exercise.

Dynamic stretches for the trunk can be done standing or sitting. Sitting position is better because it isolates joints of the trunk (vertebral column) from leg joints. Also rapid front and side bends in standing position can become ballistic stretches and harm you.

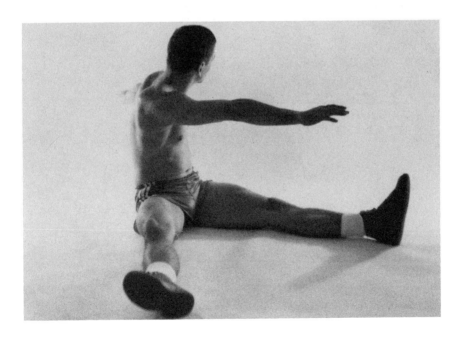

Rotations. Sit down and twist your trunk from side to side. Try to keep your hips and legs immobile.

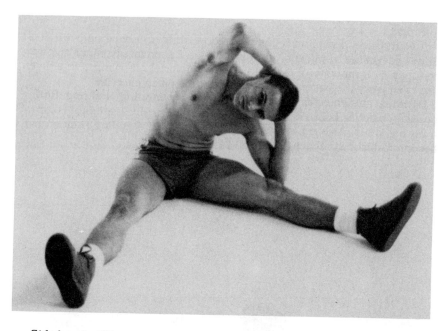

Side bends. Sitting down lean from side to side.

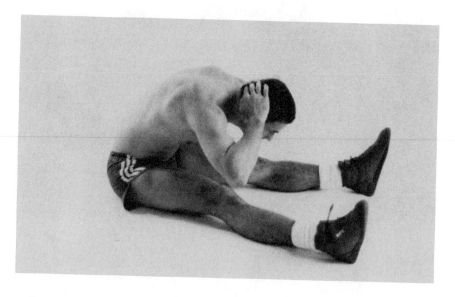

Forward bends. Lean forward from sitting position. Do not keep your back straight. Let it get round. If you keep it straight, you stretch your hamstrings.

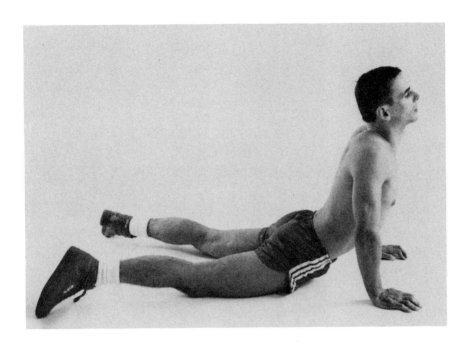

Bends to the back. Lie on your stomach and raise your trunk using your arms and muscles of the back.

Neck

Usually no special dynamic stretches are used for the neck. What you have done at the beginning of your warm-up, doing joint rotations, should be enough.

V. Static Active Flexibility Exercises

It is difficult to develop static active flexibility to the level approaching your dynamic or static passive flexibility. You have to learn how to relax stretched muscles and you have to build up strength of muscles opposing them, so parts of your body can be held in extended positions. Although this kind of flexibility requires isometric tensions to display it, you should use also dynamic strength exercises for its development. For example; training to hold your leg extended to the side, keep raising and lowering it slowly in one continuous motion. When you can do more than six repetitions add resistance (ankle weights, pulleys or rubber bands). After dynamic strength exercises, do a couple of static (isometric) exercises holding the leg up for six seconds (or longer each time) then do static passive flexibility exercises like isometric or relaxed stretches. Your static active flexibility depends on your static passive flexibility.

Exercises

You will see sets of static active flexibility exercises, each set followed by its result.

Arm extension to the back.

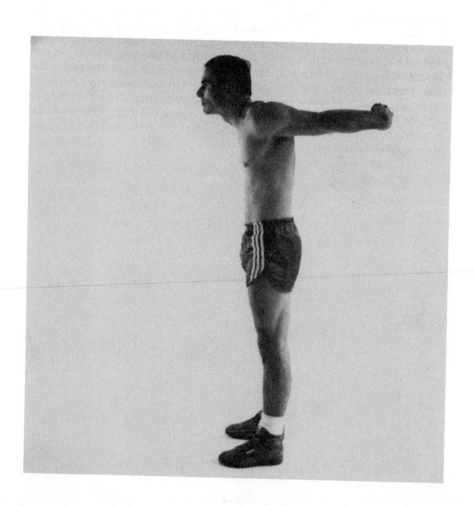

Leg extension to the front.

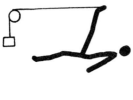

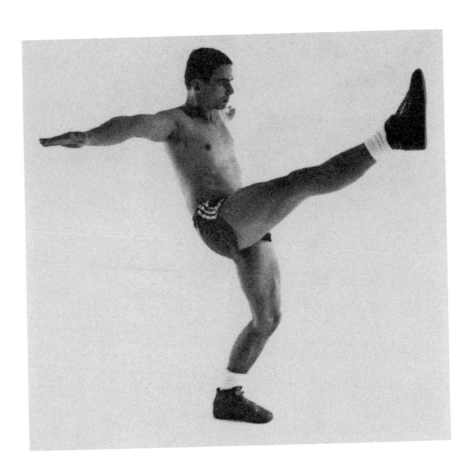

Leg extension to the side.

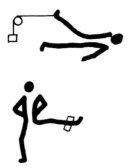

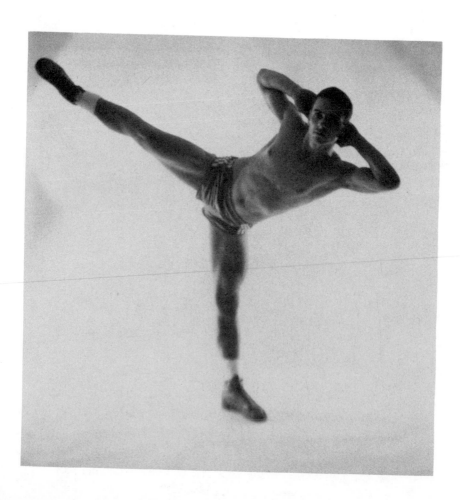

Leg extension to the back.

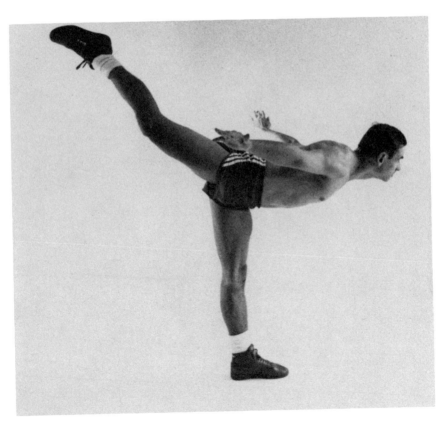

You can do all the above exercises simply, as to and fro movements, or to make them more difficult, "write" numbers or words with your foot.

Hamstring and back stretch.

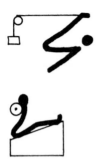

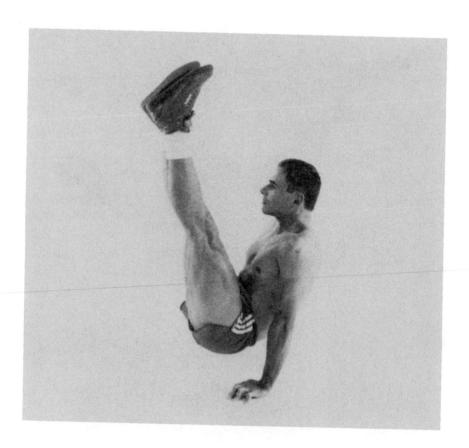

Side bend.

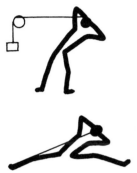

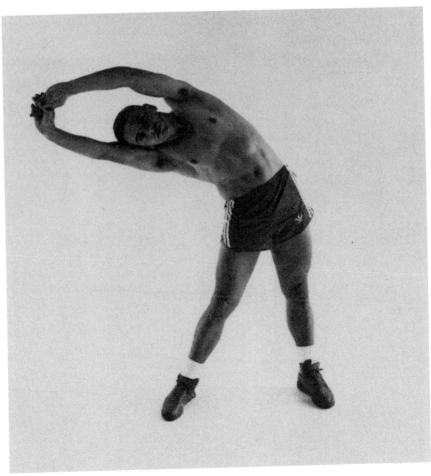

Trunk rotation.

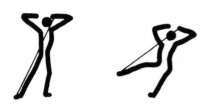

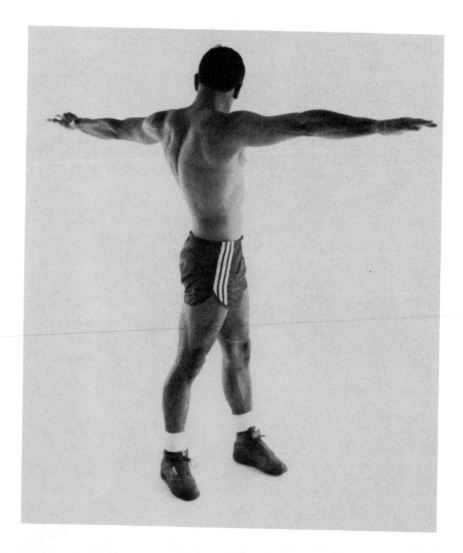

Back extension.

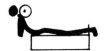

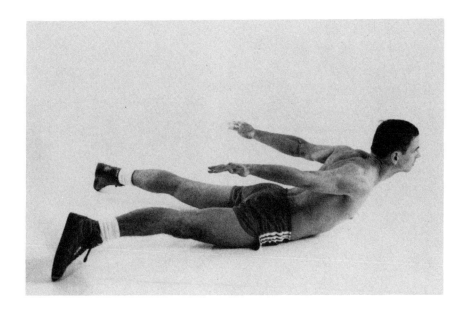

VI. Isometric Stretching

In this chapter and in the next one (Relaxed Stretching) you will learn how to develop static passive flexibility. Passive flexibility usually exceeds active (static and dynamic) flexibility in the same joint. The greater is this difference, the greater the reserve tensility (flexibility reserve) and the possibility of increasing the amplitude of active movements. This difference diminishes in training when the active flexibility improves. Doing static stretching alone does not guarantee an increase of dynamic flexibility proportional to the increase of static flexibility.

Static flexibility may increase when muscles are somewhat fatigued. This is why static stretching should be done at the end of a workout.

Isometric stretching is the fastest method of developing static passive flexibility. In isometric exercises muscle fibers contract and connective tissue attached to them is stretched. When connective tissue is stretched with too much force, it breaks down, and muscle soreness results. Soviet researchers recommend doing isometric exercises four times a week, ten to fifteen minutes per day, using tensions lasting five to six seconds. The amount of tension should increase gradually and reach maximum by third and fourth second. In particular case of isometric stretching, the last tension, applied at your maximal stretch, can be held much longer, for up to thirty seconds or sometimes even a couple of minutes. The attempt to develop strength by **isometric exercises only** may lead to stagnation of strength in six to eight weeks. To develop exceptional strength as well as flexibility, combine isometric stretches with dynamic strength exercises like lifting weights using the same muscles. After a few weeks from starting isometric stretching you may hit a plateau. Regulating the tension and length of muscles will stop bringing any improvements in your stretches. Do not worry. Do your exercises concentrating on strength gains in them. These can be expressed by increased time you can maintain a position, amount of weight you can support or ability to stand up (slide up, walk up) from your attempts at splits. After some time, when your strength improves, you will notice great increase in your flexibility.

If as a result of isometric stretching, or any other exercises, your muscles hurt, reduce the intensity of exercises or even stop working out, so you can heal completely. When the pain is gone, if isometrics (as stretches or as strength exercises) caused the problem, prepare yourself for using them again by doing normal, dynamic strength exercises gradually increasing resistance. If, for example stretching your legs by isometric stretches caused pain in any of the leg muscles, stop exercising. Wait till the pain is gone, then try marching, running, running up the incline, climbing stairs or doing squats. Do these exercises in such a way as to strengthen the injured muscles. After these exercises and at the end of regular workouts use relaxed stretches instead of isometric ones till you fully recover. Reintroduce isometrics into your training gradually, adjusting the number and strength of tensions as well as frequency in the training week to what you feel in your muscles. When everything is all right, you feel nothing—no pain, no soreness.

Recap

Isometric stretches are strenuous exercises requiring adequate rest between applications. For best results they should be supplemented by dynamic strength exercises. In the workout all dynamic exercises must precede isometrics (not counting episodic inclusion of isometric tension before speed- strength actions, which sometimes act as a stimulating factor, and in certain other cases).

Several studies have been conducted to determine the number and frequency of isometric tensions needed for greatest strength gain (increase of strength in isometric stretches means increased length of muscles). In some studies subjects using the once-per-day, 66% of maximum contraction, had results equaled by subjects using an 80% of maximum contraction performed five times per day. Another study shows greatest strength development using five to ten maximal contraction per day, five days per week. Other researchers report that using maximal contractions every other day is best. Soviet researchers recommend doing isometrics four times a week, using maximal tension held for five to six seconds, repeating each exercise three to five times.

Results shown in this chapter were obtained by following the last method and according to this plan:

Monday—technical workout followed by isometric stretches.
Tuesday—strength workout followed by isometric stretching.
Wednesday—endurance workout, no static stretching was done.
Thursday—day off.
Friday—technical training followed by isometric stretching.
Saturday—speed-strength training followed by isometric stretching.
Sunday—day off.

Usually on every first day (Monday, Friday) stretching, as well as the whole workout, was lighter than on the following day (Tuesday, Saturday). "Listening" to your body, you will be able to find the combination that works for you. Any muscle soreness or pain is a signal to stop exercises. Do not resume your training if you feel any discomfort or even a trace of pain.

Stretches

There are three methods of doing isometric stretches:

First method: Stretch the muscles (not maximally though) and wait couple of seconds till the mechanism regulating their length and tension readjusts, then increase the stretch, wait again, then stretch again. When you cannot stretch any more this way, apply short, strong tensions to bring about further increases of muscle length. Hold the last tension for up to 30 seconds.

Second method: Stretch as much as you can, hold this stretched and at the same time tensed position till you get muscle spasms, then decrease the stretch, then increase it, tense again, and so on. The last tension is held for up to five minutes. It makes some people scream.

Third method: This one was used to get the results shown in this book. Stretch the muscles nearly to the maximum, then tense for three to five seconds, then stretch further and so on, till the stretch cannot be increased. Then hold the last tension for up to 30 seconds. After a minute of rest repeat the same stretch. Do three to five repetitions of a whole stretch per workout. Use isometric stretches three or four times per week. Gradually increase time of the last tension to about 30 seconds.

In all these methods you should stress the strength gains in stretched position. When you cannot increase the stretch, concentrate on tensing harder or longer, or both. In time it will "translate" into greater stretch. To increase tension of a muscle at any given length—put more weight on it. In splits, not supporting yourself with arms will help.

No matter which method of isometric stretching you choose, when doing stretches, breathe as naturally as possible. It is not always easy with isometrics but keep trying.

Neck

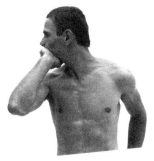

Turn your head to the side, block it with your hand and try turning it back against resistance of your arm. Relax and turn further in the same direction. Tense again. Hold the last tension for up to 30 seconds. Change side.

Stretch for muscles of the neck and the upper back (trapezius, sternocleidomastoideus, splenius capitis et cervicis, rectus capitis posterior maior, semispinalis capitis et cervicis, obliquus capitis inferior, multifidus cervicis).

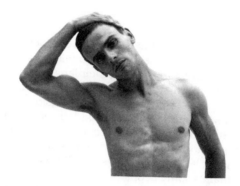

Lean your head toward the shoulder, block it with your arm, tense stretched muscles of the neck as if trying to straighten the head. Relax and bring it closer to the shoulder. Tense again. Hold the last tension for up to 30 seconds. Change side.

Stretch for muscles of the neck and the upper back (sternocleidomastoideus, splenius capitis, scalenus anterior, scalenus medius, scalenus posterior, splenius cervicis, longissimus capitis, levator scapulae).

Forearm

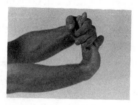

Bend your wrist. Hold your hand, tense, relax, flex more. Hold the last tension for up to 30 seconds. Change hands.

Stretch for muscles flexors of the hand (flexor carpi radialis, palmaris longus, flexor carpi ulnaris, flexor digitorum sublimis, flexor digitorum profundus).

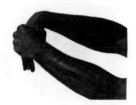

Bend your wrist in opposite direction. Tense, relax, flex again. Hold the last tension for up to 30 seconds. Change hands.

Stretch for muscles extensors of the hand (extensor carpi radialis longus, extensor carpi radialis brevis, extensor digitorum communis, extensor carpi ulnaris).

Arms, Shoulders, Chest.

These stretches are for tennis players, swimmers, gymnasts, basketball players, team handball players, golfers, discus and javelin throwers and hockey players. Students of certain martial arts (Indian muki boxing, wushu, sambo) requiring great mobility of shoulders will find these exercises useful. Judoka, sambo wrestlers, cyclists, skaters and hockey players can use stretches #1 and #4 as corrective exercises for rounded back.

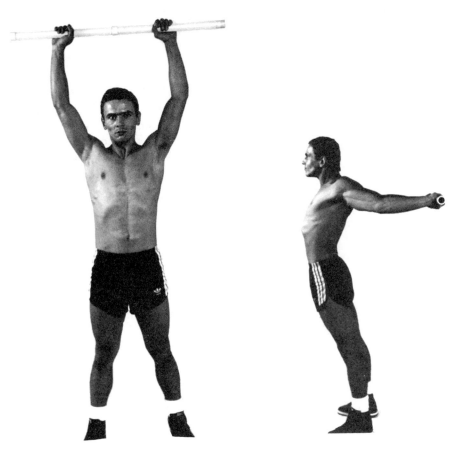

#1. Starting from this position, bring the stick to the position behind your back, tense all the stretched muscles, relax, bring the stick to the front, make your grip narrower, bring the stick to the back and tense again. When the grip is so narrow that you cannot lower your arms any more—stop and tense stretched muscles for up to 30 seconds. This exercise stretches front of the arms, shoulders and the chest (pronator teres, palmaris longus, brachioradialis, biceps brachii, coracobrachialis, deltoideus, pectoralis maior, pectoralis minor, teres maior, serratus anterior, subscapularis).

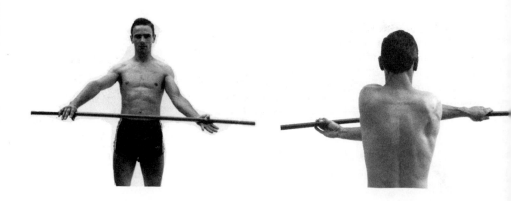

#2. Change the grip. Twist the stick. Tense your upper back, shoulders and triceps. Relax. Move your hands further apart on the stick. Twist it again and tense stretched muscles. Hold the last tension for up to 30 seconds. Stretch for the muscles of the upper back (trapezius, rhomboideus, latissimus dorsi).

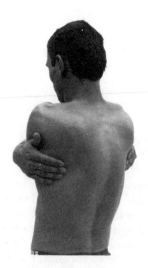

#3. Variation of the previous stretch. Crawl your hands as far on your back as you can.

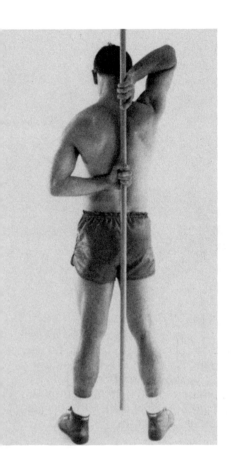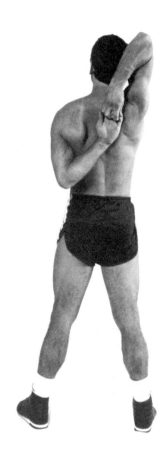

#4. Through successive tensions and relaxations crawl your hands toward each other. Hold the last tension for up to 30 seconds. Switch position of hands. Stretch for muscles of arms, shoulders, chest and upper back (triceps, anconeus, deltoideus, pectoralis maior, latissimus dorsi, teres maior, supraspinatus).

Legs
Stretches leading to the side split. Useful to martial artists, soccer players, skiers, hurdlers, dancers, skaters, gymnasts, judoka and sambo wrestlers.

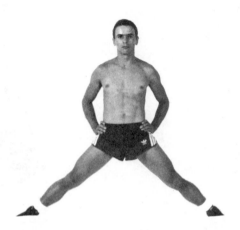

Tense inside of your thighs as if trying to "pinch" the floor. Relax, spread the legs further. Keep repeating the cycle of tensions and relaxation till you cannot lower yourself any more without pain. Hold the last tension for up to 30 seconds. Doing this exercise do not lean forward and do not support yourself with your arms. The trunk should be kept straight. Get out of the stretch without using your arms. Stretch for muscles of the inner thigh (adductor magnus, adductor brevis, adductor longus, gracilis, pectineus).

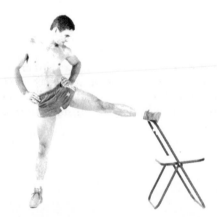

Another version of the previous stretch. Gradually increase the height of support or the distance from supporting leg to the support. In the latter case use something stable and not too high, for example a pile of gymnastic pads, as your support.

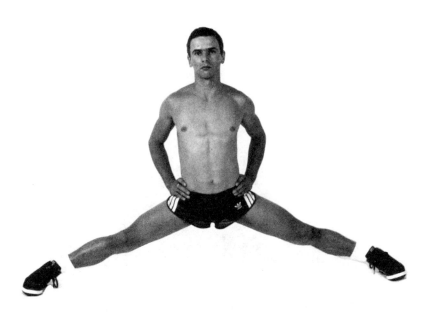

To get from this position to the full side split it should take you about one month. At this stage people with weak knees may experience problems. In such cases strength exercises for the muscles stabilizing the knees will help.

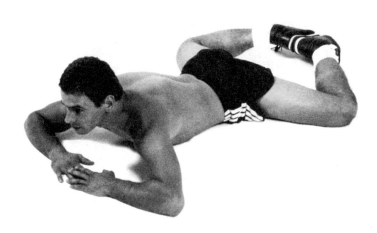

Here is an exercise you can do instead of previous ones should you have any knee problems. General principle is the same as usual—try "pinching" the floor with your knees and alternate tensions and relaxations to get your hips as low as possible.

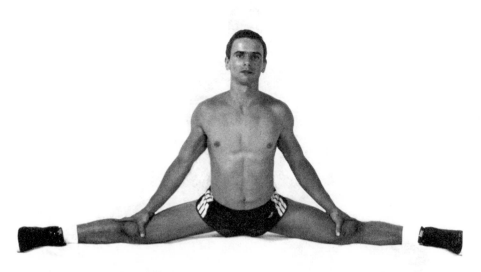

Full side split. Spend 30 seconds or more in this position tensing inside of your thighs. Try lifting yourself off the floor by sheer strength of your legs. Eventually you should be able to slide up from the split to standing position without using your arms. Then you can try full side split in suspension.

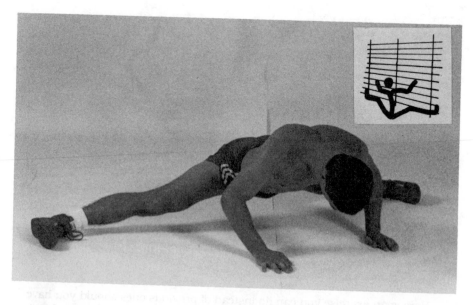

Exercises for different kind of side split—side split with toes pointing upward. Stretches for the muscles described on page 64 and muscles of the buttocks (gluteus medius and gluteus minimus).

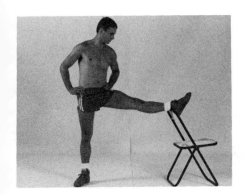 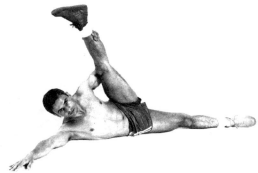

Two more versions of the previous stretch.

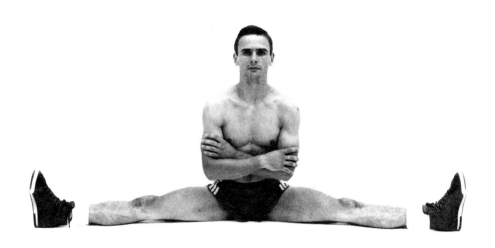

Side split with toes pointing upward.

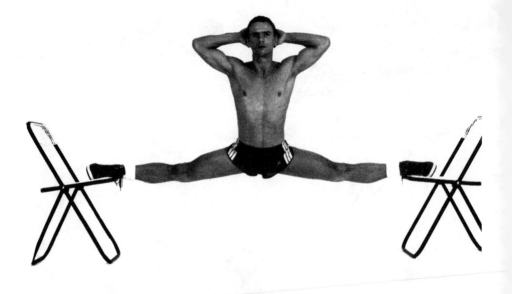

Full side split in suspension. Be careful. Loss of balance may put your muscles out of commission for a year or more. First attempts should be done on objects low enough so you can rest on the floor without tearing muscles should you lose your balance.

Stretches leading to the front split. Important for cyclists, dancers, gymnasts, skaters, skiers, track and field athletes, wrestlers, judoka, sambo wrestlers and martial artists.

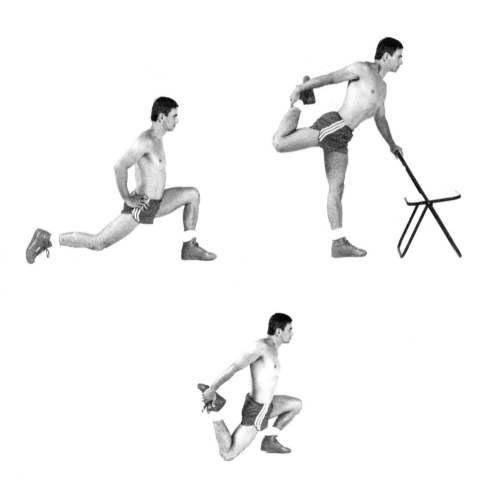

Tense muscles that bring your thigh forward and straighten your knee. Relax, stretch, tense again. Hold the last tension for up to 30 seconds. Change sides. These are the stretches for muscles that bring the thigh up, i.e., in running, and the muscles that straighten the knee (iliacus, psoas maior, rectus femoris, vastus lateralis, vastus medialis, vastus intermedius, sartorius, adductor magnus, adductor longus, adductor brevis, tensor fasciae latae, obturatorius internus, gracilis, gluteus minimus, pectineus).

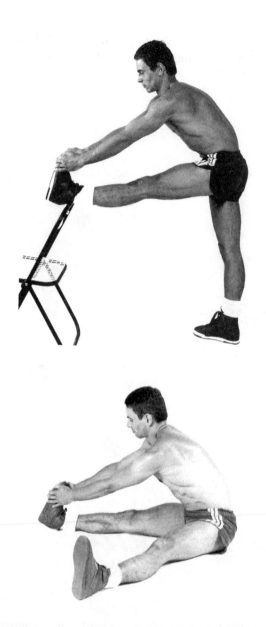

Calf pull. Grab and pull your toes toward yourself. Point your foot forward against resistance of your arms. Relax, pull the toes closer to yourself and start pointing the foot forward again. Hold the last tension for up to 30 seconds. Change legs. Stretch for muscles of the calf (gastrocnemius, soleus, plantaris, flexor hallucis longus, tibialis posterior, flexor digitorum longus, peroneus longus, peroneus brevis).

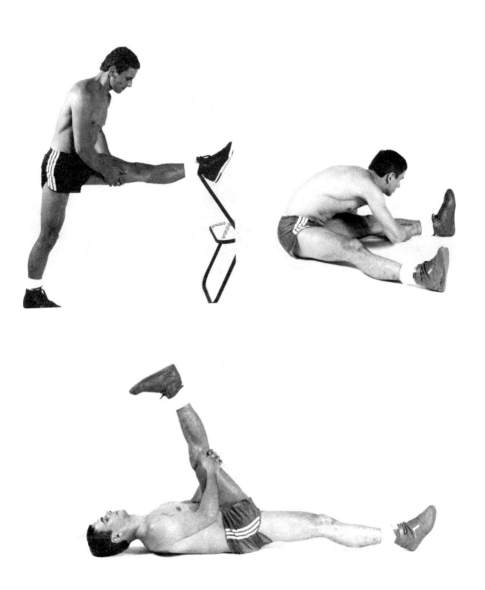

Hamstring stretch. Using either one of the shown positions stretch your hamstring increasing the angle between your thighs. Tense the hamstring, relax it and either pull your leg toward yourself or if using support, move supporting leg further back. Tense again, relax and stretch more. Hold the last tension for up to 30 seconds. Change the leg. Stretch for hamstrings, buttocks and some of the pelvic muscles (biceps femoris, semimembranosus, semitendinosus, adductor magnus, gluteus maximus, gluteus medius, piriformis, obturatorius internus).

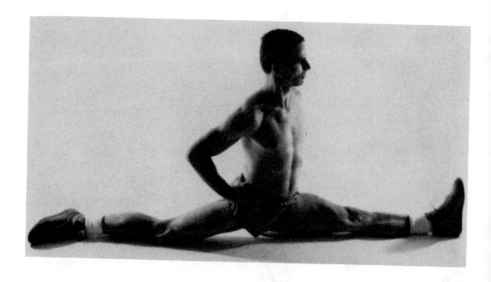

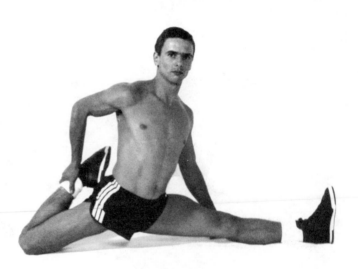

Pinch the floor tensing hamstring of your front leg, quadriceps and the so called runners muscles of the rear leg. Relax, lower your hips. Tense again. Hold the last tension for up to 30 seconds. Change side. Stretch for muscles of thighs, buttocks and pelvis (iliacus, psoas maior, rectus femoris, vastus lateralis, vastus medialis, vastus intermedius, sartorius, adductor magnus, adductor longus, adductor brevis, tensor fasciae latae, obturatorius internus, gracilis, gluteus minimus, pectineus).

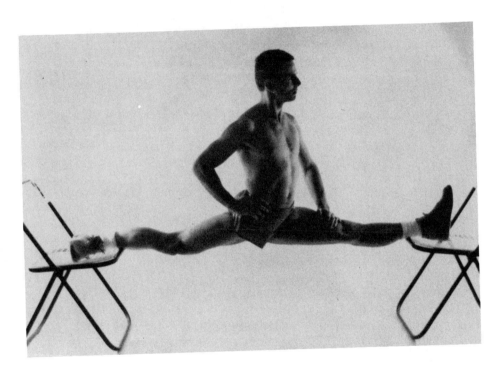

Full front split in suspension.

Trunk

Stretches for track and field athletes (throwers), wrestlers, judoka, gymnasts, dancers, tennis players.

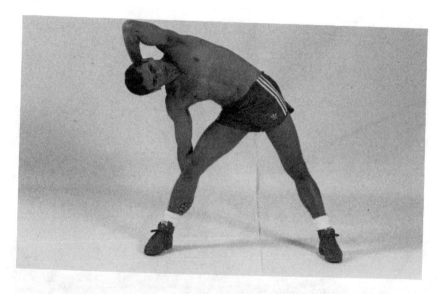

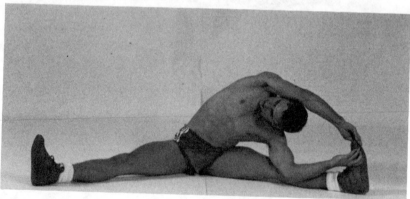

Side bends. Do not twist or lean forward. Move only to the side. Tense the stretched side, relax and try leaning further to the side. Hold the last tension for up to 30 seconds. Change sides. Stretch for muscles of the side of abdomen and of the back (quadratus lumborum, longissimus dorsi, iliocostalis, obliquus abdominis externus, obliquus abdominis internus, psoas maior).

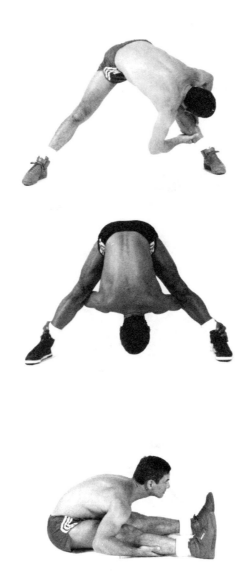

Lower back and hamstring stretch. Grab your legs and tense your back as if trying to straighten up. Relax, lean forward and tense again. Keep your head straight. Hold the last tension for up to 30 seconds.

Stretch for muscles of the back, buttocks and hamstrings (longissimus, iliocostalis, multifidus, gluteus maximus, gluteus medius, adductor magnus, biceps femoris, semitendinosus, semimembranosus, piriformis, obturatorius internus), and muscles of the calves.

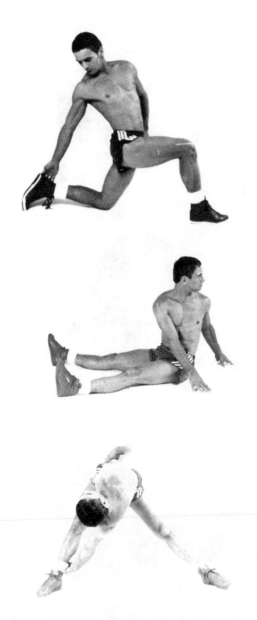

Trunk rotation. Twist (rotate) your trunk, grab your foot or put your hands on the ground, tense stretched muscles of your trunk, relax and twist further. Tense again, relax, stretch and hold the last tension for up to 30 seconds. Change sides. Stretch for muscles of the back and the abdomen (semispinalis, multifidus, mm. rotatores, obliquus abdominis externus, obliquus abdominis internus).

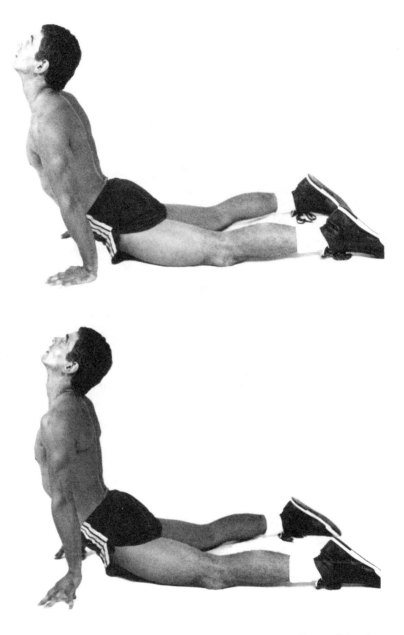

Abdomen stretch. Tense your abdomen as if trying to pull your hips forward and down. Relax, lower your hips and tense again. Hold the last tension for up to 30 seconds. Stretch for front of the abdomen, muscles on front of the spine and inside the pelvis (rectus abdominis, obliquus abdominis externus, obliquus abdominis internus, quadratus lumborum, psoas maior, psoas minor).

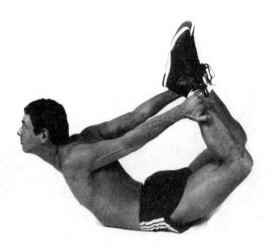

More intensive version of previous stretch affecting also front of thighs. Usually your lower back will get very tense while you do these abdomen stretches. You can even get cramps. To relax the back, do any of the following "counterstretches". They can be done without tensing.

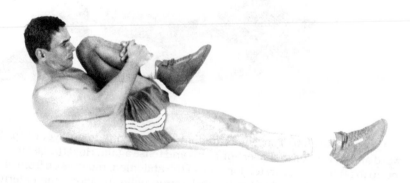

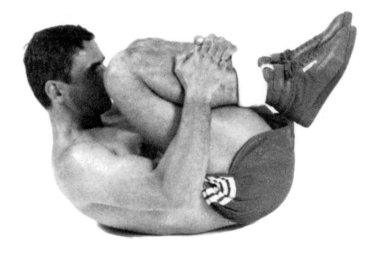

Remember—a partner in stretching can cause an injury. If you need some-
one's help in doing any stretches, it means that you are not ready for them.
Rather go slow but steady.

VII. Relaxed Stretching

Relaxed stretches are yet another means of developing static passive flexibility. Although much slower than isometric stretches, relaxed stretches have some advantages over isometrics. They do not cause fatigue and you can do them when you are tired. It is hard to get any problem doing them. Two major drawbacks; muscular strength in extended positions does not increase as a result of relaxed stretching and are they slow . . . For the same person, that using isometrics gets into a full side split in 30 seconds without a warm-up, it may take even ten minutes of relaxed stretching, also with no warm-up, to get there. Within a couple of months of doing relaxed stretches this time gets shorter. Eventually it may take you from one to two minutes to do a full split. (With good warm-up, of course, you can do it at once.) In your workout relaxed stretches should be done as the last thing. Do them after isometric stretches or instead of them. If you have enough time in a day, you can also do them, without a warm-up, whenever you feel like it.

Doing these stretches assume positions that let you relax all muscles. Remember isometric stretches? Some of their positions are designed to tense stretched muscles, e.g., side and front split exercises, by placing your weight on them. In relaxed stretching you want as little weight on your muscles as possible. In splits it is done by leaning the body forward and supporting it with arms. Relax completely. Think about slowly relaxing all muscles. Do not think about anything energetic or unpleasant. Relaxing into a stretch, at some point, you will feel resistance. Wait in that position patiently and after a while you will notice that you slide into a new range of stretch. After reaching greatest possible stretch (greatest at this stage of training), hold it feeling mild pain in stretched muscles. Get out of the stretch after a minute or two. Do not stay in a stretch till you get muscle spasms. You can repeat the stretch after a minute.

Relaxed stretches

Neck

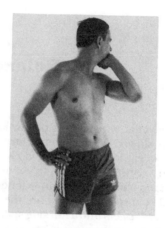

Put your hand on your cheek or your chin. Turn your head to the side. Use your hand to increase range of motion.

Muscles stretched: trapezius, sternocleidomastoideus, splenius capitis et cervicis, semispinalis capitis et cervicis, rectus capitis posterior maior, obliquus capitis inferior, multifidus cervicis.

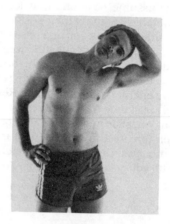

Put your hand on the side of your head. Lean your head toward the shoulder. Use your hand to increase the stretch.

Muscles stretched: sternocleidomastoideus, splenius capitis, scalenus anterior, scalenus posterior, iliocostalis cervicis, splenius cervicis, longissimus capitis, levator scapulae.

Forearm

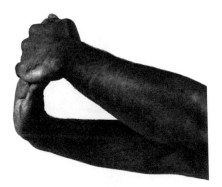

Bend your wrist using your other hand to increase the stretch.
Stretch for muscles flexors of the hand (flexor carpi radialis, palmaris longus, flexor carpi ulnaris, flexor digitorum sublimis, flexor digitorum profundus).

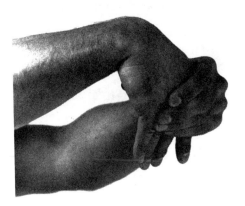

Bend your wrist in opposite direction using your other hand to increase the stretch.
Stretch for muscles extensors of the hand (extensor carpi radialis longus, extensor carpi radialis brevis, extensor digitorum communis, extensor carpi ulnaris).

Arms, Shoulders, Chest.

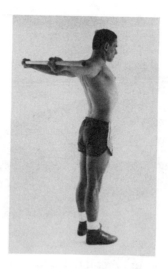

Bring the stick to the position behind your back, using the narrowest grip possible.

Stretch for muscles of the front of the arms, shoulders and the chest (biceps brachii, pronator teres, palmaris longus, brachioradialis, coracobrachialis, deltoideus, pectoralis maior, serratus anterior, subscapularis).

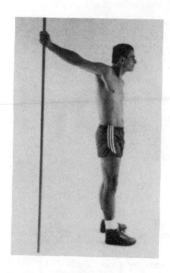

You can stretch the same muscles doing this stretch.

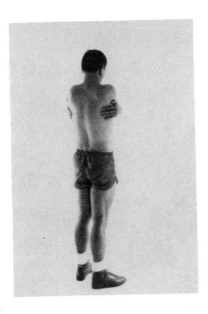

Change grip on the stick and twist it.
Stretch for muscles of the upper back (trapezius, rhomboideus, latissimus dorsi).

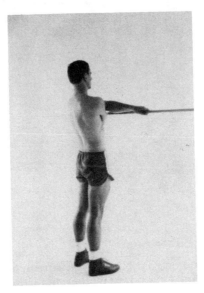

Another form of upper back stretch.
Crawl your hands on your back as far as you can.

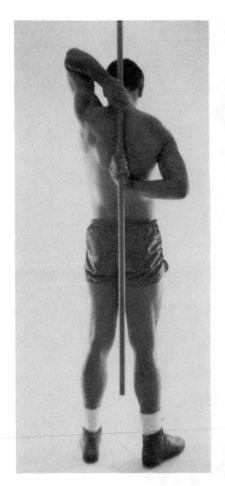 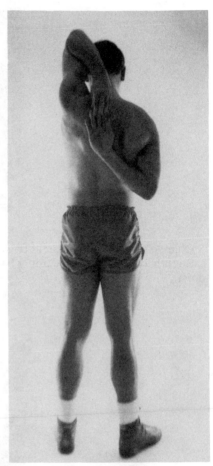

Grab your hands behind your back. If you cannot, use a piece of rope or a stick to crawl your hands toward each other. In turns, pull down the upper hand, then pull up the lower hand to feel a good stretch.

Muscles stretched: triceps, anconeus, deltoideus, pectoralis, latissimus dorsi, teres maior, supraspinatus.

Legs

Exercises leading to the side split.

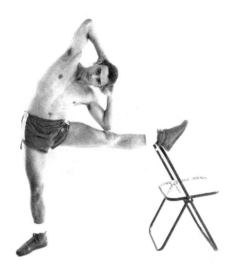

Place your leg on any support. Either lean toward this leg or move the other leg away from the support.

You can also lift your leg with your hand.

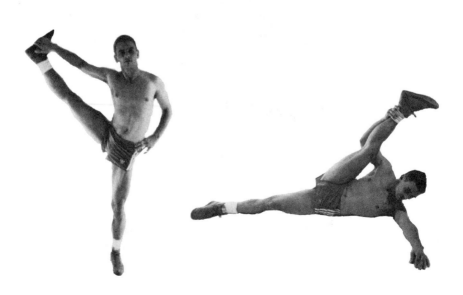

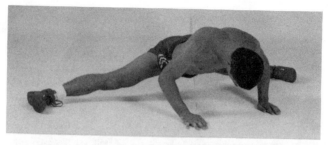

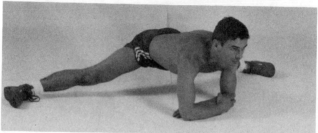

Stretch muscles of the both inner thighs in this position. Shift your weight between your legs and arms to get the best stretch. When legs tense, help them relax putting most of your weight on the arms. When the legs relax, slide into greater stretch shifting the weight back.

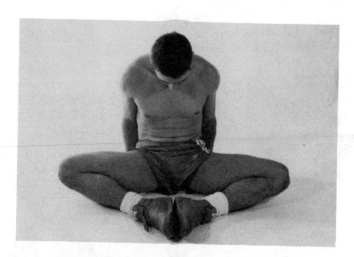

One more, even milder inner thigh stretch. Sit down, bend your knees and pull your feet together. Now, lower the thighs using only strength of muscles that abduct and rotate them externally. Do not push with hands.

Stretches for muscles of the inner thigh (adductor magnus, adductor brevis, adductor longus, gracilis, pectineus).

Exercises leading to the front split.

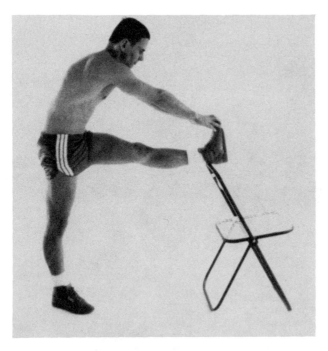

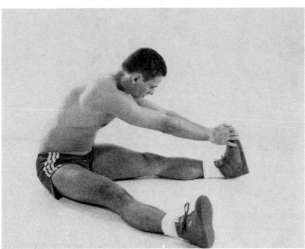

Calf stretches. Pull your toes toward yourself. Feel stretching in muscles of the calf (gastrocnemius, soleus, plantaris, flexor hallucis longus, tibialis posterior, flexor digitorum longus, peroneus longus, peroneus brevis).

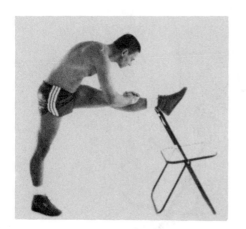 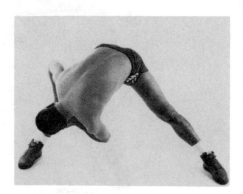

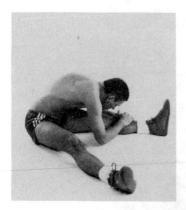 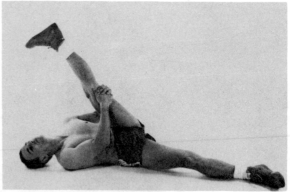

Hamstring stretches. Using any of the shown positions stretch your hamstrings.

Muscles stretched: biceps femoris, semimembranosus, semitendinosus, adductor magnus, gluteus maximus, gluteus medius, piriformis, obturatorius internus.

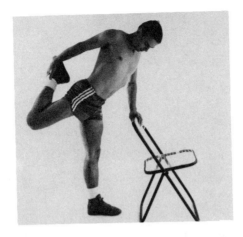

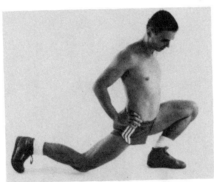

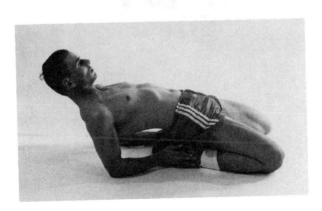

Quadriceps stretches. These are stretches for muscles of the front of the thigh and the so called runner's muscles originating inside the pelvis and in front of the spine(iliacus, psoas maior, rectus femoris, vastus lateralis, vastus medialis, vastus intermedius, sartorius, adductor longus, adductor brevis, tensor fasciae latae, obturatorius internus, adductor magnus,gracilis, gluteus minimus, pectineus).

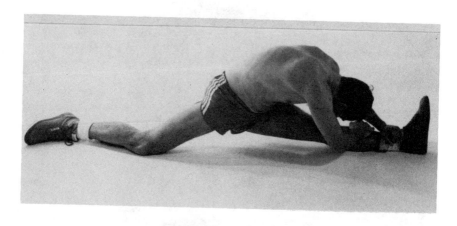

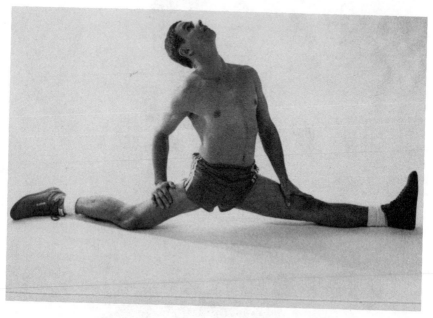

Sit in the split. Lean your trunk forwards and backwards to stretch all the muscles of the thigh, buttocks and the pelvis.

Muscles stretched: iliacus, psoas maior, rectus femoris, vastus lateralis, vastus medialis, vastus intermedius, sartorius, adductor magnus, adductor longus, adductor brevis, tensor fasciae latae, obturatorius internus, gracilis, gluteus maximus, gluteus medius, gluteus minimus, pectineus, biceps femoris, semimembranosus, semitendinosus, piriformis.

Trunk

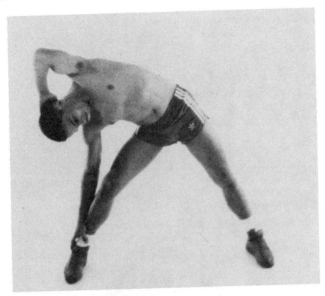

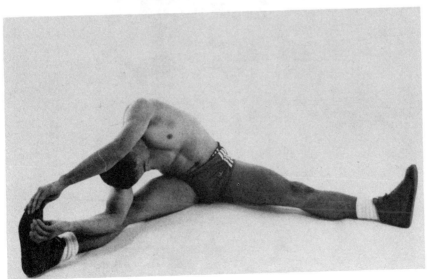

Side bends. Bend your trunk to the side. Do not twist or lean your trunk forward.

Stretch for the muscles of the back and the side of the abdomen (quadratus lumborum, longissimus dorsi, iliocostalis, obliquus abdominis internus, obliquus abdominis externus, psoas maior).

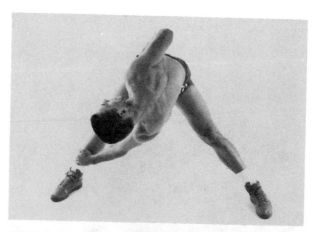

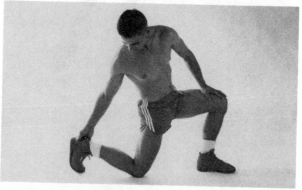

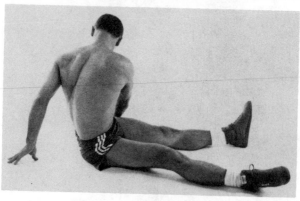

Trunk rotations. Rotate your trunk as far as it takes to feel a mild stretch. You can increase the stretch and then help yourself keep it using the hand on your leg or on the floor.

Muscles stretched: obliquus abdominis externus, obliquus abdominis internus, semispinalis, multifidus, mm. rotatores.

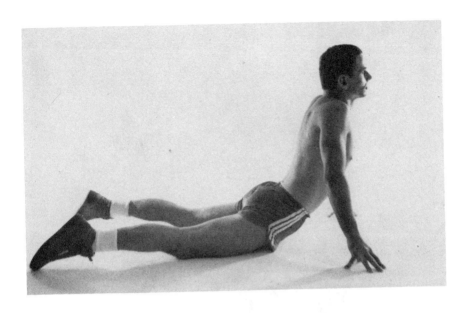

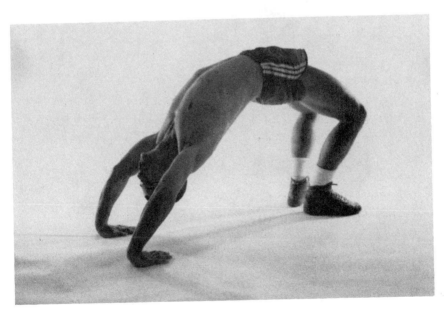

Abdomen stretches. Stretches for front of the abdomen and the muscles on front of the spine and inside the pelvis (rectus abdominis, obliquus abdominis externus, obliquus abdominis internus, quadratus lumborum, psoas maior, psoas minor).

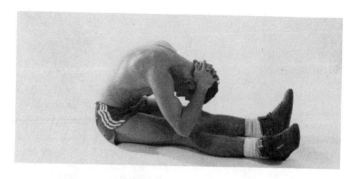

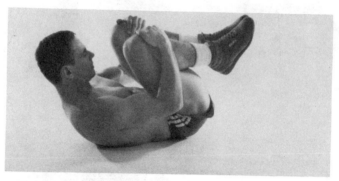

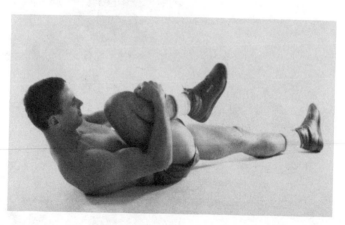

Lower back stretch. Stretch as much as it takes to relax the muscles of the back and not to stretch its ligaments. Stretching ligaments of the back weakens it. This is why I do not show a relaxed stretch for the back in a standing position. The weight of the upper body hanging on your relaxed spine can stretch its ligaments. To feel stretching in the muscles of your back, arch it. Keeping back straight stretches your hamstring.

Muscles stretched: longissimus dorsi, iliocostalis, multifidus.

VIII. Sample Workout Plans

Here you get examples of how to choose exercises depending on the task of your workout and when to do them in the course of the workout. I picked several disciplines of sport. Each is represented by one workout with the task common for that discipline. These are just the examples and not prescriptions. In professionally run training process no workout is the same. Each workout has either different task or the task is realized by different means every time. Different tasks and different means of their realization are assigned to workouts depending on the age, class and condition of the athletes. Planning workout the coach has to take into consideration workouts done thus far, the next tasks that need to be done, when the athletes need their form to peak and much more. To put it simply: your skill level and condition change from workout to workout, and so do your exercise needs.

In the following examples I show only the flexibility exercises related to the task of the workout. The exercises of the main part of the workout are not shown.

Discipline: Track and Field—Hurdles. Task of the workout: Technique of passing the hurdles. No work on the start from the blocks or on the finish.

General warm-up.

Jogging with rotations of the joints

March with knee raises.

March with leg raises to the front

March with leg raises to the side

Specific warm-up.

March with passing hurdles.

Main part.

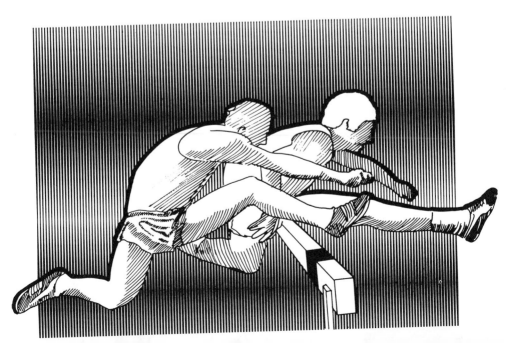

Cool-down.

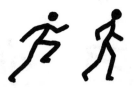

Jogging.   March with lunges.

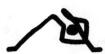

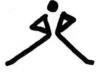

Isometric stretches.

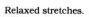

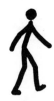

Relaxed stretches.   March.

Discipline: Gymnastics. Task of the workout: Development of flexibility and perfection of the handstand (this task is usually realized with children nine to ten years old).

General warm-up.

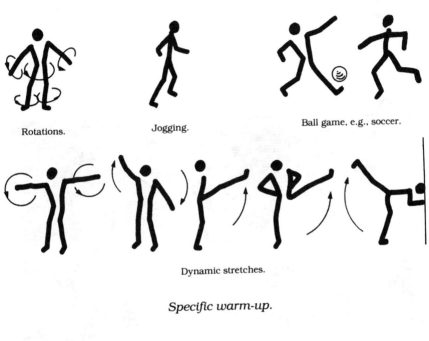

Rotations.   Jogging.   Ball game, e.g., soccer.

Dynamic stretches.

Specific warm-up.

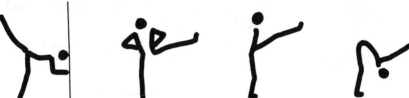

Static active flexibility exercises.

Relaxed stretches.

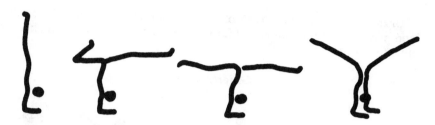

Forearm stand.   Splits in forearm stand.

Main part.

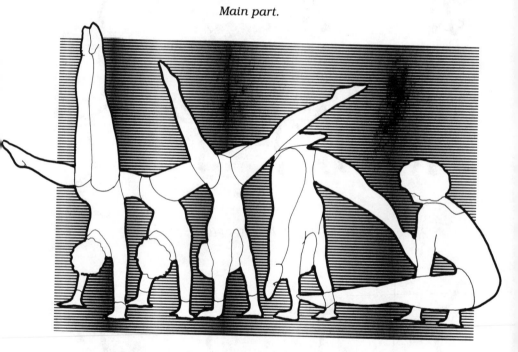

Cool-down.

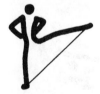 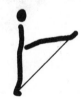

Static active flexibility exercises.

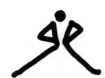 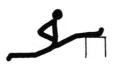

Isometric stretches.

March.

Discipline : Kickboxing. Task of the workout: High roundhouse kick.

General warm-up.

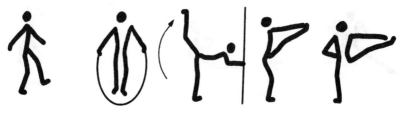

March with rotations
of the joints

Jumping rope.

Dynamic stretches.

Specific warm-up.

Knee kicks.

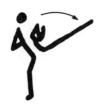

Roundhouse kicks

Main part.

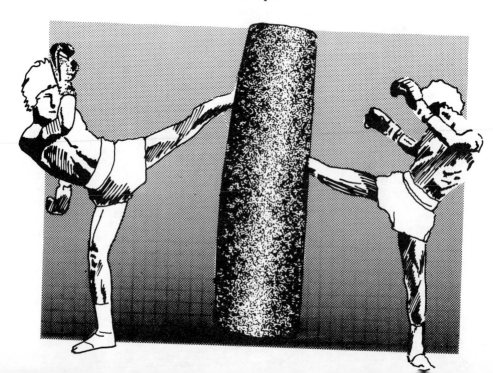

Cool-down.

Front lunges.

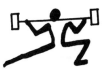

Side lunges.

Isometric stretches.

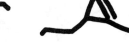

Relaxed stretches.

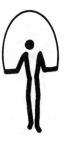

Jumping rope.

Discipline: Judo. Task of the workout: Teaching O-Soto-Gari (big outside sweep).

General warm-up.

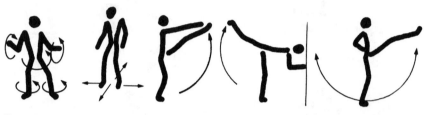

Rotations
of the joints

Judo steps.

Dynamic stretches.

Leg swings.

Specific warm-up and the main part of workout

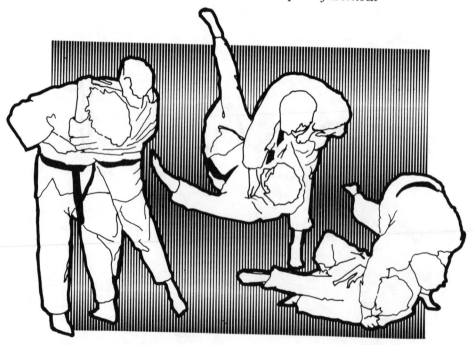

Cool-down.

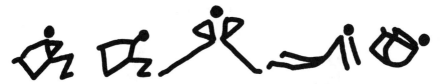

Isometric stretches.

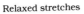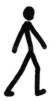

March.

Relaxed stretches

Discipline: Bodybuilding. Task of the workout: Developing strength of the upper back, chest, forearms and lower legs.

General warm-up.

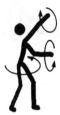 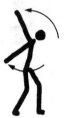

March with rotations of the joints.   Dynamic stretches.

Specific warm-up and the main part of workout

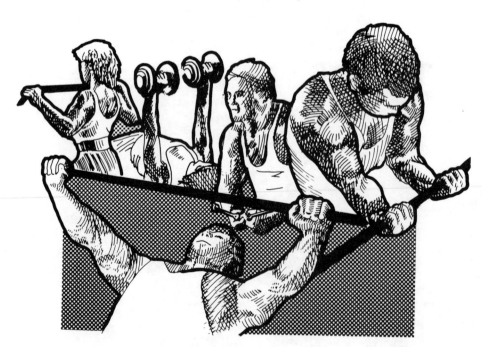

Cool-down.

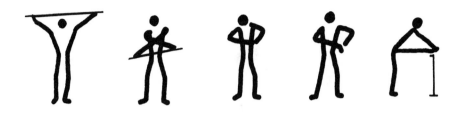

Relaxed stretching.

Discipline: Swimming. Task of the workout: Speed in butterfly stroke.

General warm-up.

 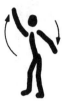 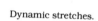

Rotations of the joints.   Dynamic stretches.

Specific warm-up, main part and most of the cool-down in the pool.

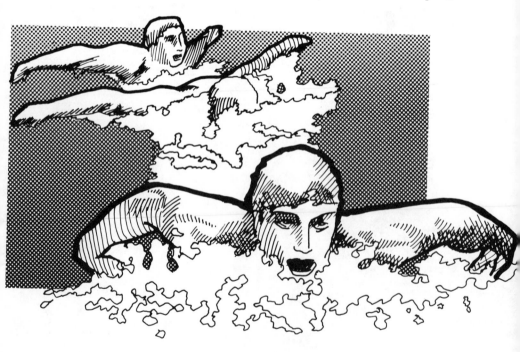

Cool-down.

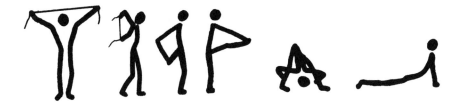

Relaxed stretches.

Appendix: Normal Range of Joint Motion

Neck
Flexion 70-90 degrees. . . . . Touch sternum with chin.
Extension 55 degrees. . . . . Try to point up with chin.
Lateral bending 35 degrees . . . . Bring ear close to shoulder.
Rotation 70 degrees left & right . . . . Turn head far to the left, then right.

Lumbar Spine
Flexion 75 degrees. . . . . Bend forward at the waist.
Extension 30 degrees . . . . Bend backward.
Lateral bending 35 degrees . . . . Bend to the side.

Shoulder
Abduction 180 degrees. . . . . Bring arm sideways up.
Adduction 45 degrees . . . . Bring arm toward the midline of the body.
Horizontal extension 45 degrees . . . . Swing arm horizontally backward.
Horizontal flexion 130 degrees . . . . Swing arm horizontally forward.
Vertical extension 60 degrees. . . . . Raise arm straight backward.
Vertical flexion 180 degrees . . . . Raise arm straigth forward.

Elbow
Extension 180 degrees . . . . Straighten out lower arm.
Flexion 150 degrees . . . . Bring lower arm to the biceps.
Supination 90 degrees . . . . Turn lower arm so palm of the hand faces up.
Pronation 90 degrees. . . . . Turn lower arm so palm faces down.

Wrist
Flexion 80-90 degrees. . . . . Bend wrist so palm nears lower arm.
Extension 70 degrees . . . . Bend wrist in opposite direction.
Radial deviation 20 degrees. . . . . Bend wrist so thumb nears radius.
Ulnar deviation 30-50 degrees . . . . Bend wrist so small finger nears ulna.

Hip
Flexion 110-130 degrees . . . . Flex knee and bring thigh close to abdomen.
Extension 30 degrees . . . . Move thigh backward without moving pelvis.
Abduction 45-50 degrees . . . . Swing thigh away from midline.
Adduction 20-30 degrees . . . . Bring thigh toward and across the midline.
Internal rotation 40 degrees . . . . Flex knee. Swing lower leg away from midline.
External rotation 45 degrees . . . . Flex knee. Swing lower leg toward midline.

Knee
Flexion 130 degrees . . . . Touch calf to hamstring.
Extension 15 degrees . . . . Straighten out knee as much as possible.
Internal rotation 10 degrees . . . . Twist lower leg toward midline.

Ankle
Extension 20 degrees . . . . Bend ankle so toes point up.
Flexion 45 degrees. . . . . Bend ankle so toes point down.
Pronation 30 degrees . . . . Turn foot so the sole faces in.
Supination 20 degrees. . . . . Turn foot so the sole faces out.

Bibliography

Stanislaw Grochmal. Teoria i metodyka cwiczen relaksowo- koncentrujacych. Warszawa: PZWL, 1979.

Stanislaw Borowiec, Alexander Ronikier. Zarys anatomii funkcjonalnej narzadow ruchu. Warszawa: WAWF, 1977.

Ulatowski T. Teoria i metodyka sportu. Warszawa: WAWF, 1979.

Naglak Z. Trening sportowy—teoria i praktyka. Warszawa: PWN, 1979.

Chrominski Z. Metodyka sportu dzieci i mlodziezy: Warszawa: Sport i Turystyka, 1980.

Matveyev L.P. Osnovy sportivnoy trenirovki. Moskva: Fizkultura i Sport, 1977.

Kukushkin G.I. (General Editor). Sistiema fizichieskovo vospitania v SSSR. Moskva: Raduga, 1983.

Giesielievich B.A.(editor). Medicinskii spravochnik trieniera. Moskva: Fizkultura i Sport, 1976.

deVries H.A. Physiology of Exercise for Physical Education and Athletics. Dubuque: Wm.C. Brown Company Publishers, 1980.

Bullock J., Boyle J., Wang M.B., Ajello R.R. Physiology. Media: Harval Publishing Co., 1984.

Fox E.L. Sports Physiology. Philadelphia: Saunders College Publishing, 1979. Bishop B. Basic Neurophysiology. Garden City: Medical Examination Publishing Co., Inc., 1982.

Wolf J.K. Practical Clinical Neurology. Garden City: Medical Examination Publishing Co., Inc., 1980.

Roberts T.D.M. Neurophysiology of Postural Mechanisms. Boston: The Butterworth Group, 1978

Knuttgen H.G. Neuromuscular Mechanisms for Therapeutic and Conditioning Exercise. Baltimore: University Park Press, 1976.

Russe/Gerhardt/King. An Atlas of Examination, Standard Measurements and Diagnosis in Orthopedics and Traumatology. Baltimore: The Williams and Wilkins Co., 1972.

MacConail M.A., Basmajian J.V. Muscles and Movements, a basis for human kinesiology. Baltimore: The Williams and Wilkins Co., 1969.

Breit N.J. The effects of body position and stretching technique on the development of hip and back flexibility. Dissertation for degree of Doctor of Physical Education. Springfield College, 1977.

Burkett L.N. Causative factors in hamstring strains. Master of Arts thesis. San Diego State College, 1968.

Johns R. J., Wright V. Relative importance of various tissues in joint stiffness. Journal of Applied Physiology 17:824-28, 1962.

Leighton J.R. A study of the effect of progressive weight training on flexibility. American Corrective Therapy Journal 18(4):101, 1964.

Wickstrom R.L. Weight training and flexibility. Journal of Health, Physical Education and Recreation 34(2):61, 1963.

The Hip Society. St. Louis: The C.V. Mosby Company, 1973.

Licht S.(editor). Therapeutic Exercise. Baltimore: Waverley Press, Inc., 1965.

Potter P.A. Pocket Nurse Guide to Physical Assessment. St. Louis: The C.V. Mosby Company, 1985.

Knots M., Voss D.E. PNF Patterns and Techniques. New York: Harper & Row, 1968.

INDEX